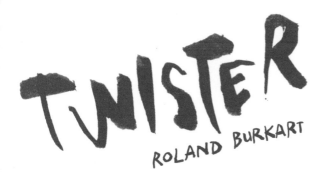

TWISTER

ROLAND BURKART

graphic mundi

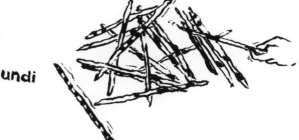

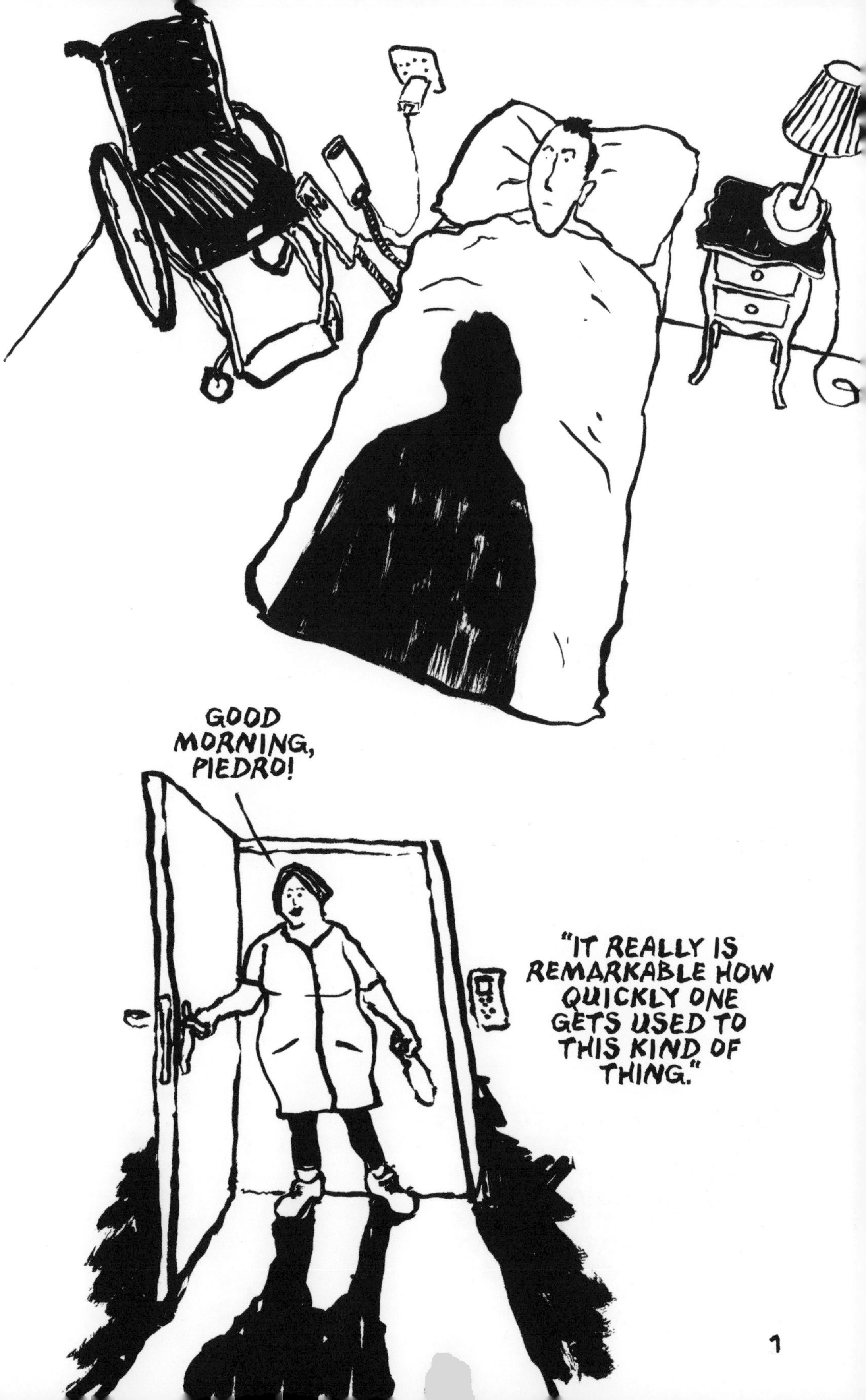
GOOD MORNING, PIEDRO!
"IT REALLY IS REMARKABLE HOW QUICKLY ONE GETS USED TO THIS KIND OF THING."

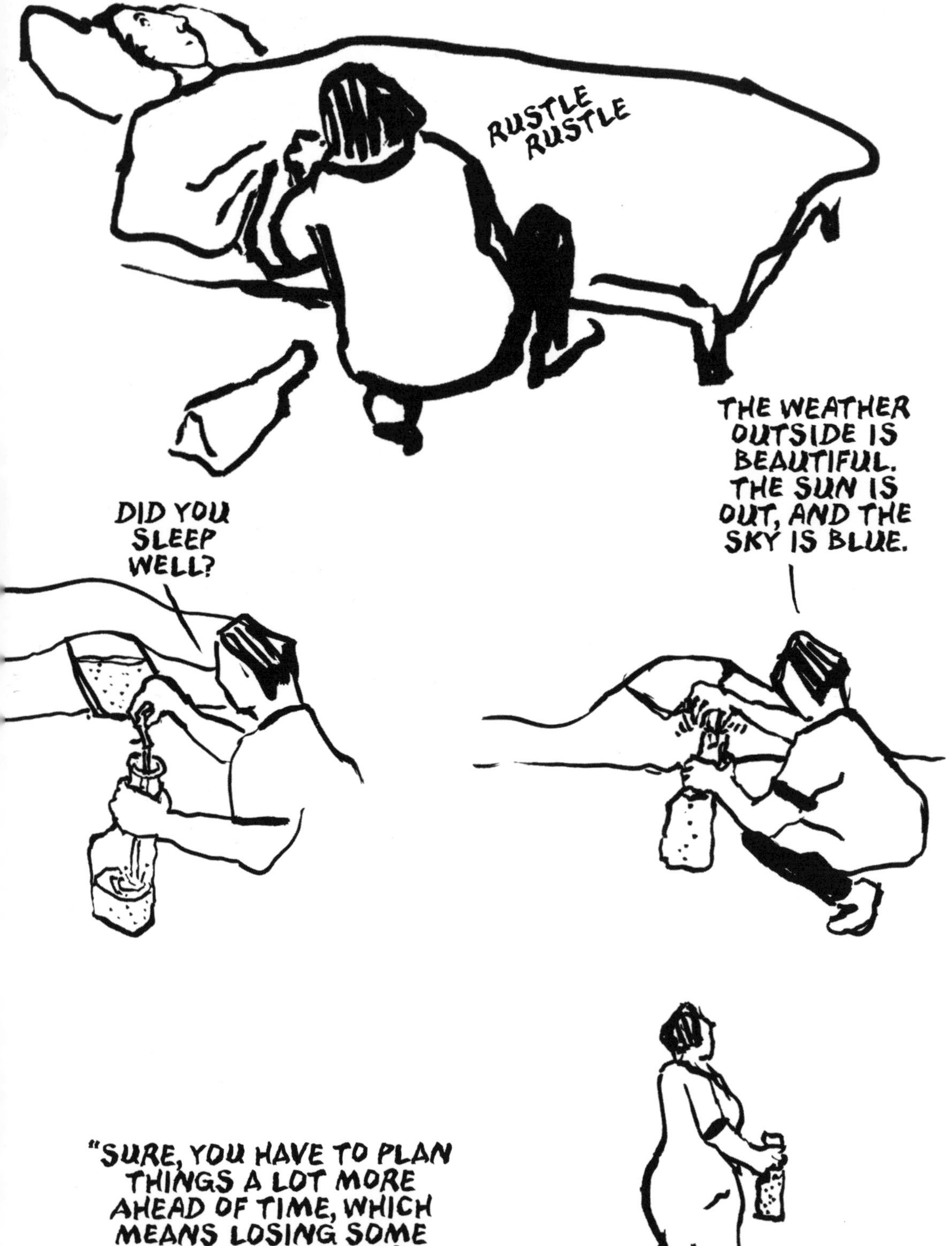
RUSTLE RUSTLE
DID YOU SLEEP WELL?
THE WEATHER OUTSIDE IS BEAUTIFUL. THE SUN IS OUT, AND THE SKY IS BLUE.
"SURE, YOU HAVE TO PLAN THINGS A LOT MORE AHEAD OF TIME, WHICH MEANS LOSING SOME SPONTANEITY. BUT I'VE BECOME MORE PATIENT. THAT WASN'T THE CASE BEFORE."

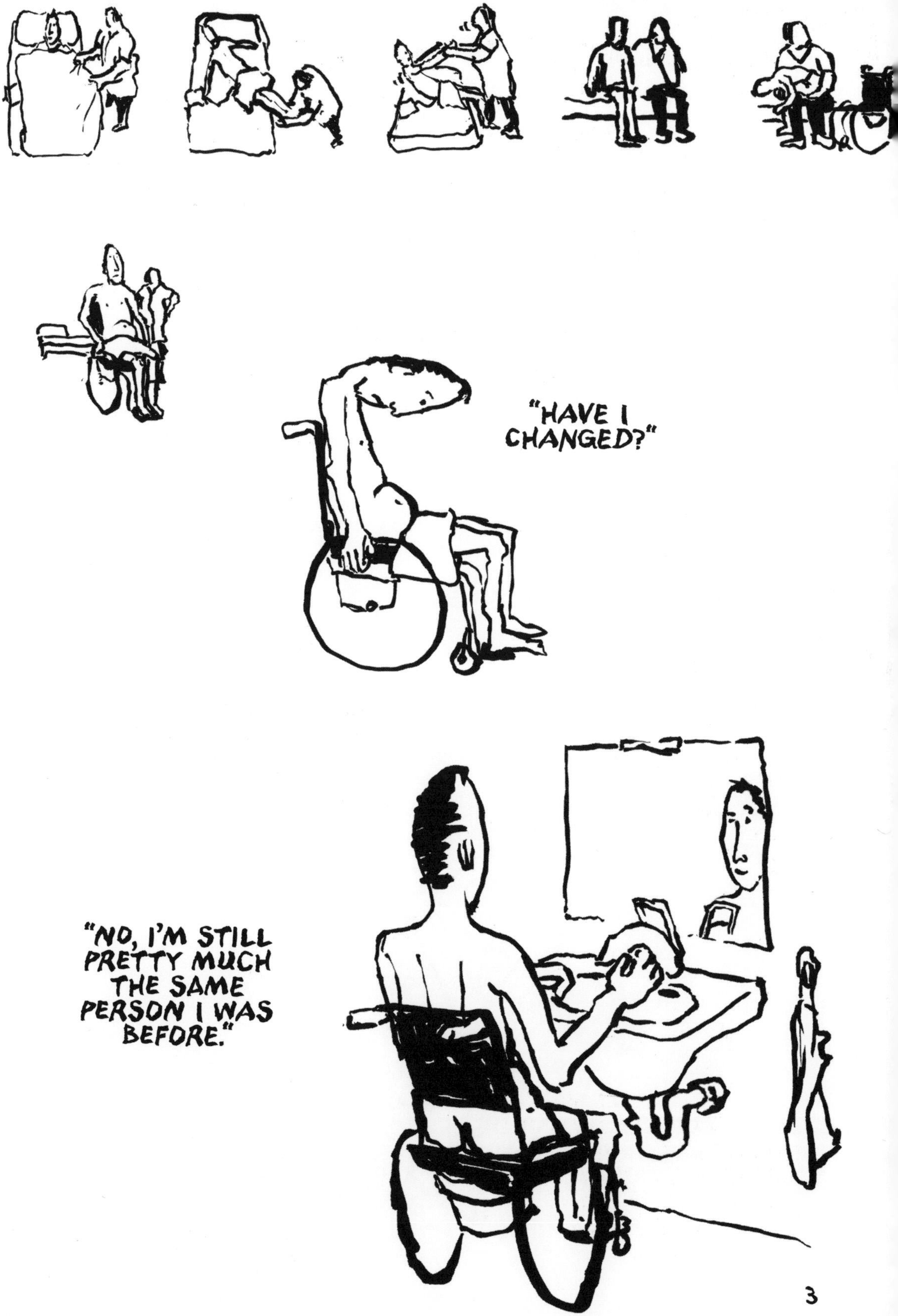
"HAVE I CHANGED?"
"NO, I'M STILL PRETTY MUCH THE SAME PERSON I WAS BEFORE."

"IT HAPPENED ON MAY 28, ALMOST THIRTEEN YEARS AGO."
BRRRRRRRRRRRRRRRRAAMMMM

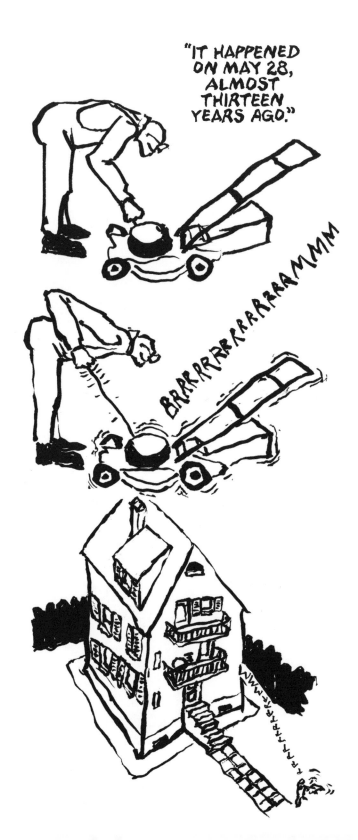

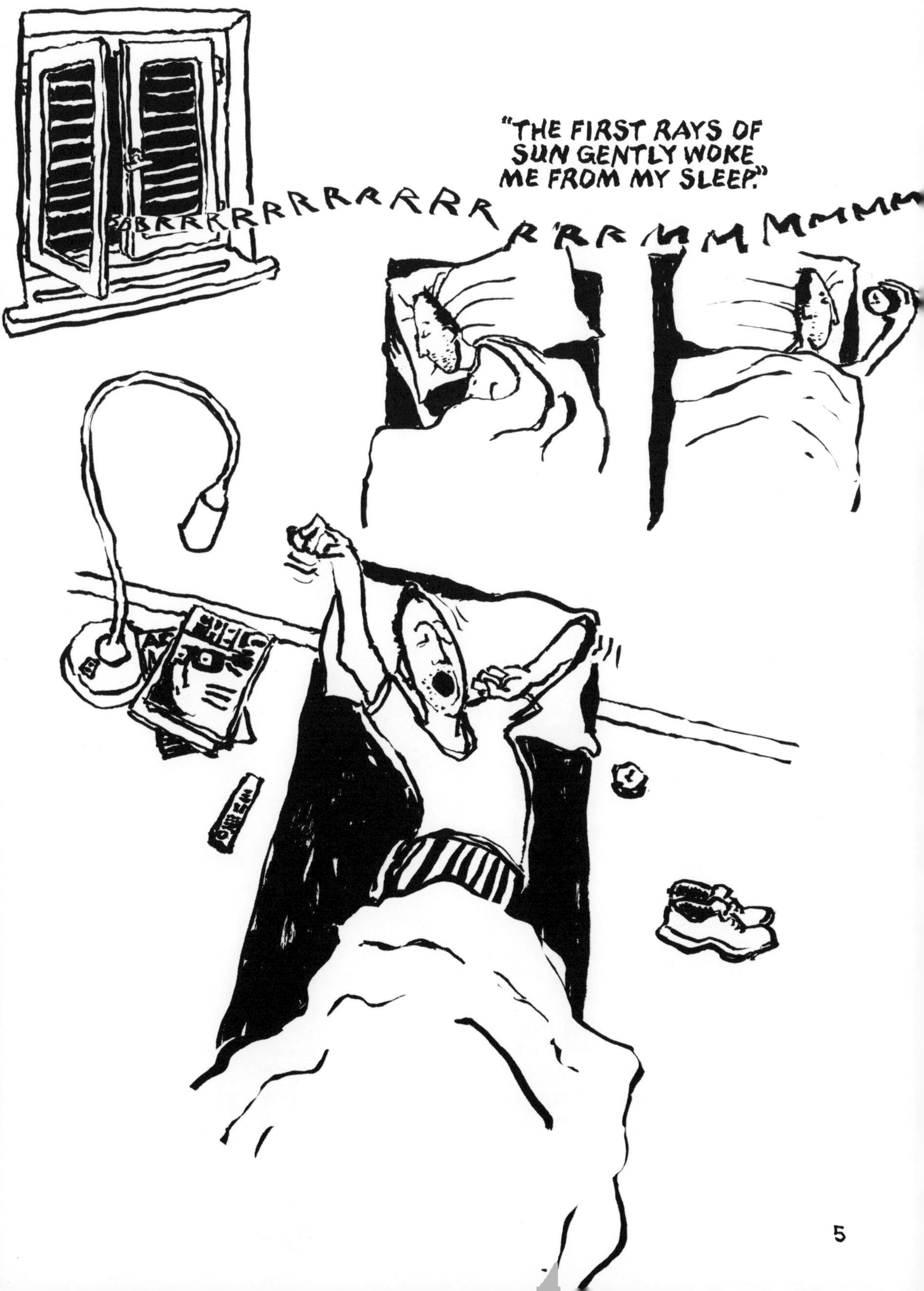
"THE FIRST RAYS OF SUN GENTLY WOKE ME FROM MY SLEEP."
BBBRRRRRRRRRRRRRRRRRRMMMMMMM

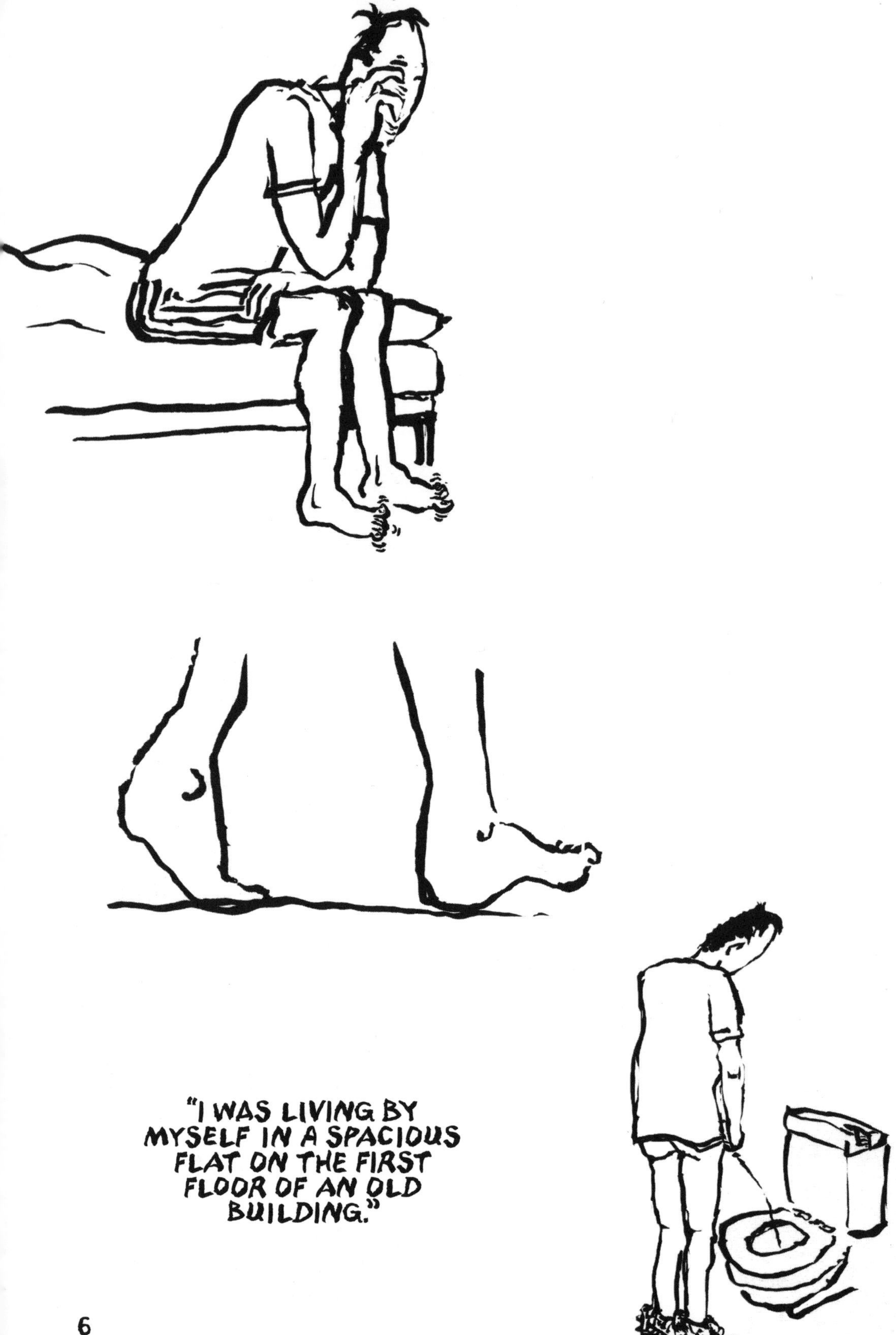
"I WAS LIVING BY MYSELF IN A SPACIOUS FLAT ON THE FIRST FLOOR OF AN OLD BUILDING."

"AS A SALES REPRESENTATIVE FOR THE FOOD MANUFACTURER 'CHICO,' I COULD AFFORD THAT."

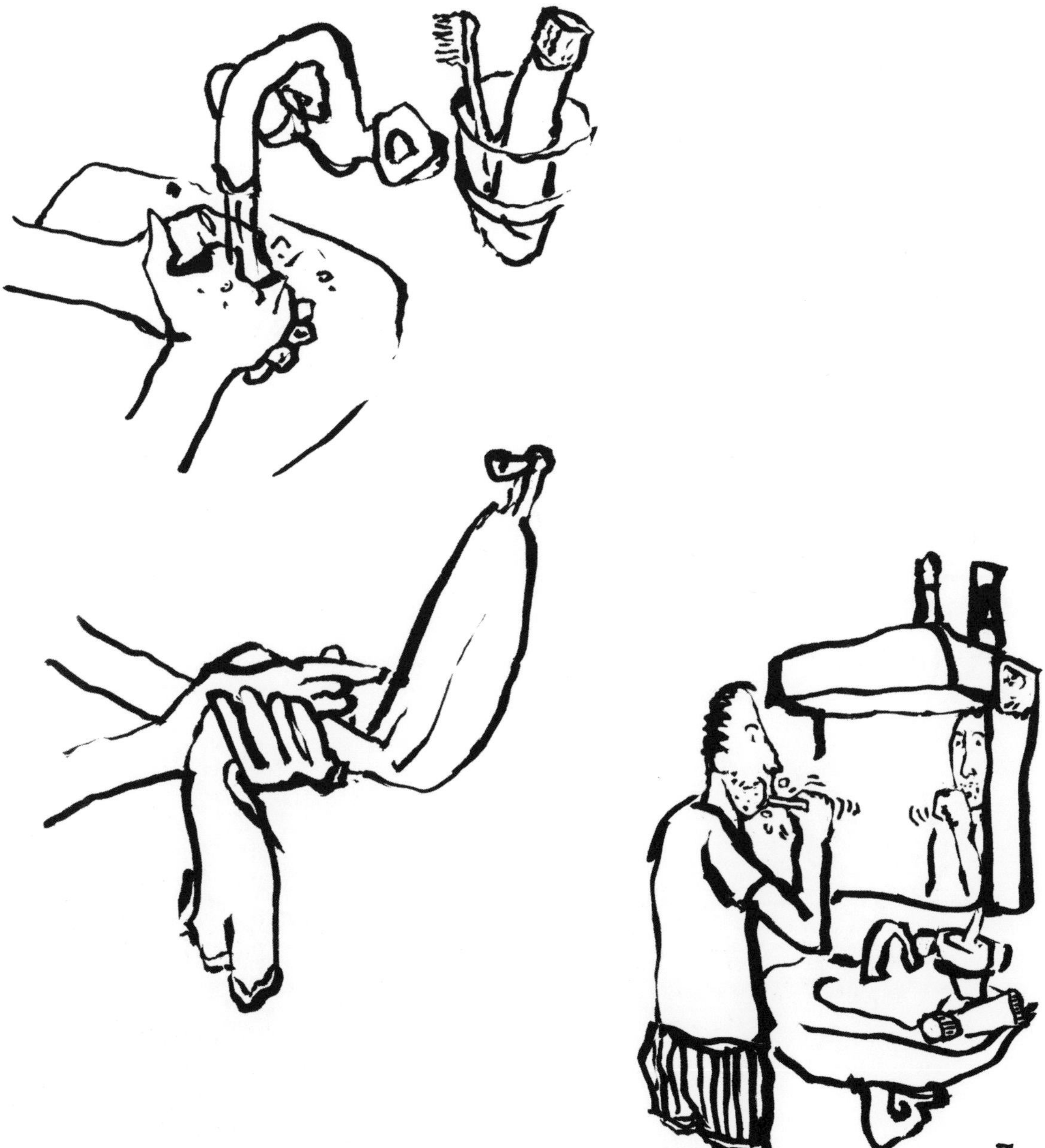

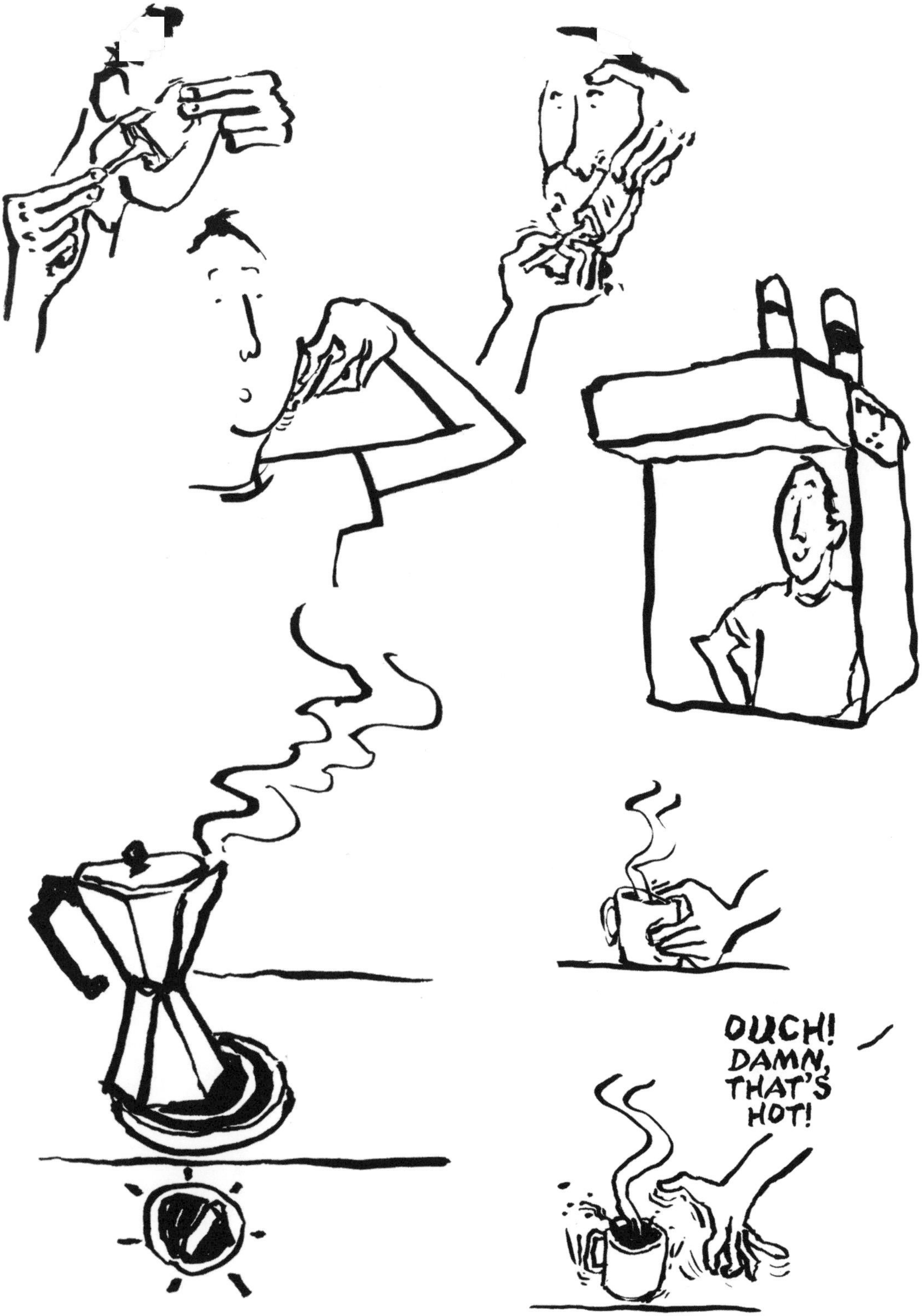
OUCH! DAMN, THAT'S HOT!

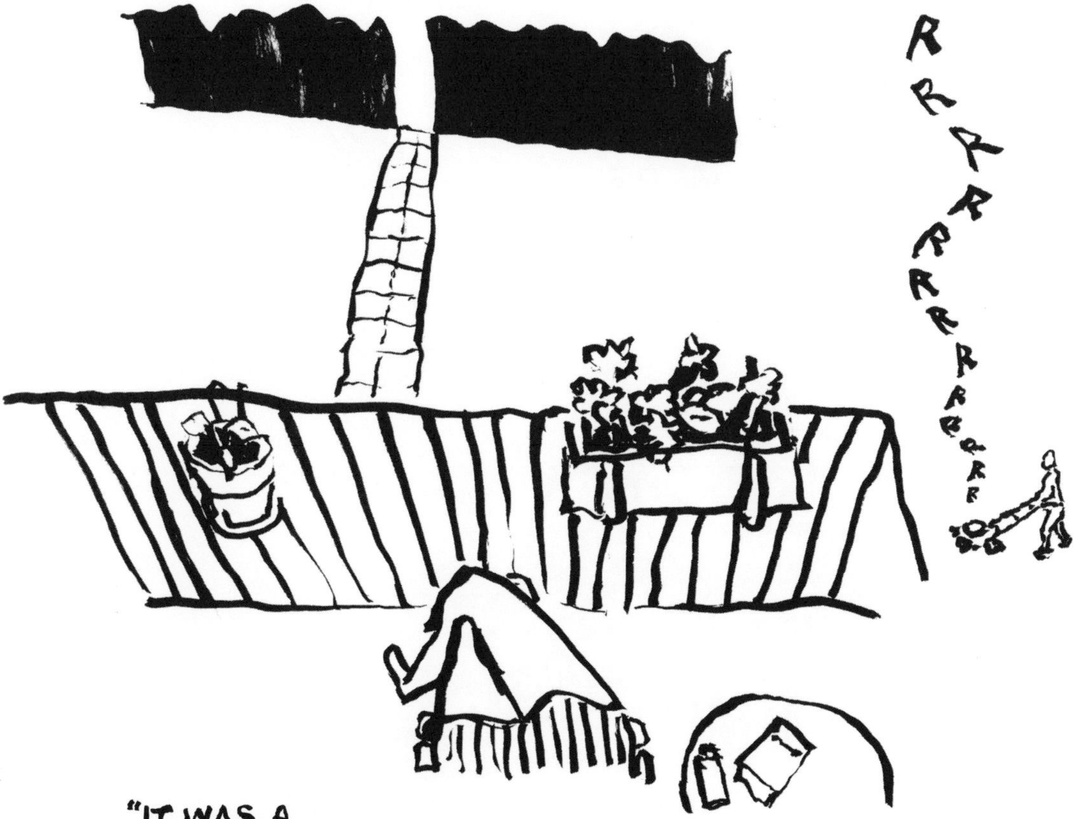
RRRRRRRRRRRRR

"IT WAS A SATURDAY, AND I WAS LOOKING FORWARD TO MY WEEKEND OFF."

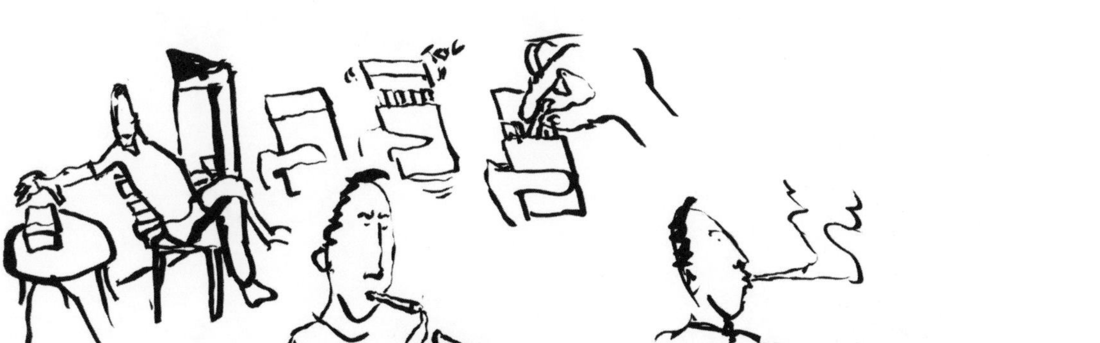

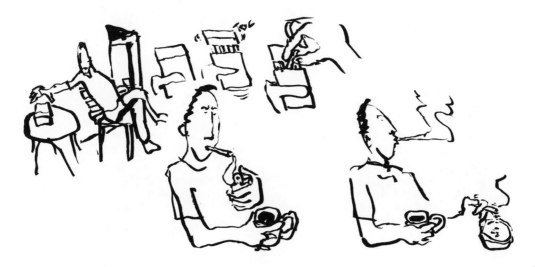

"LUCAS AND I WERE PASSIONATE SWIMMERS. WE OFTEN MET UP AT KORALLSEE ON WARM DAYS. AS WE DID ON MAY 28."

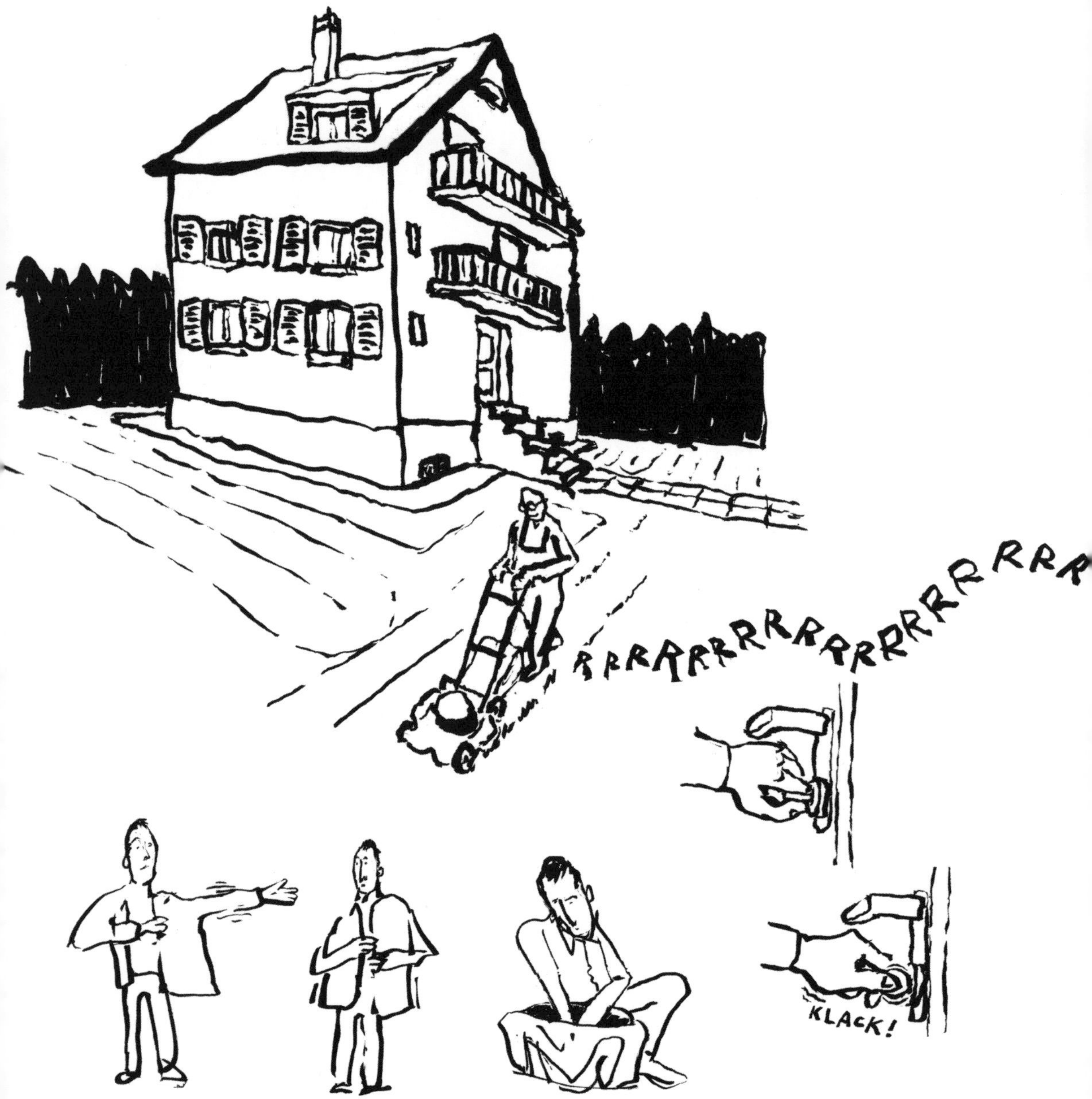
RRRRRRRRRRRRRRRRRRRRRR
KLACK!

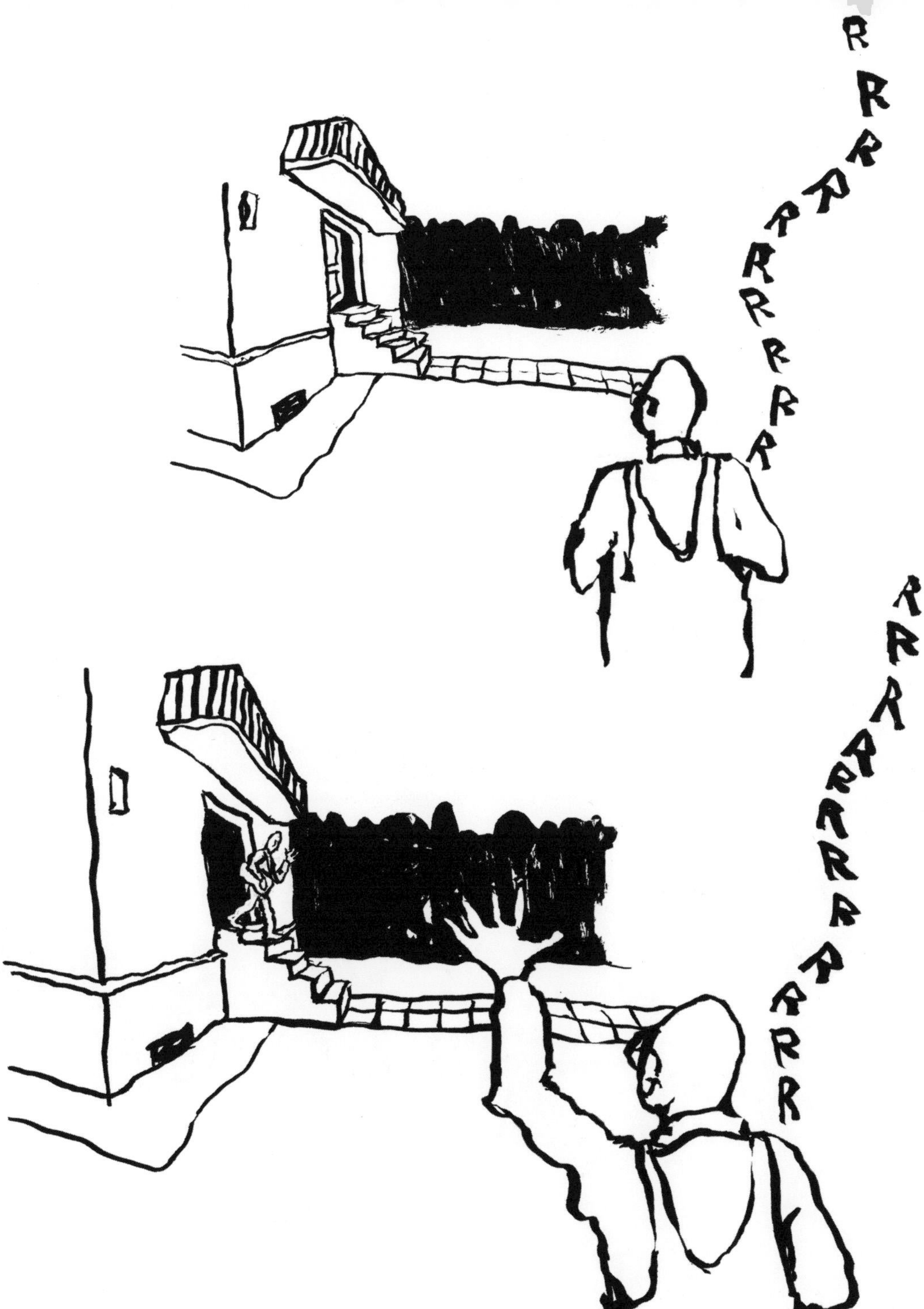
RRRRRRRRRR
RRRRRRRRRRRR

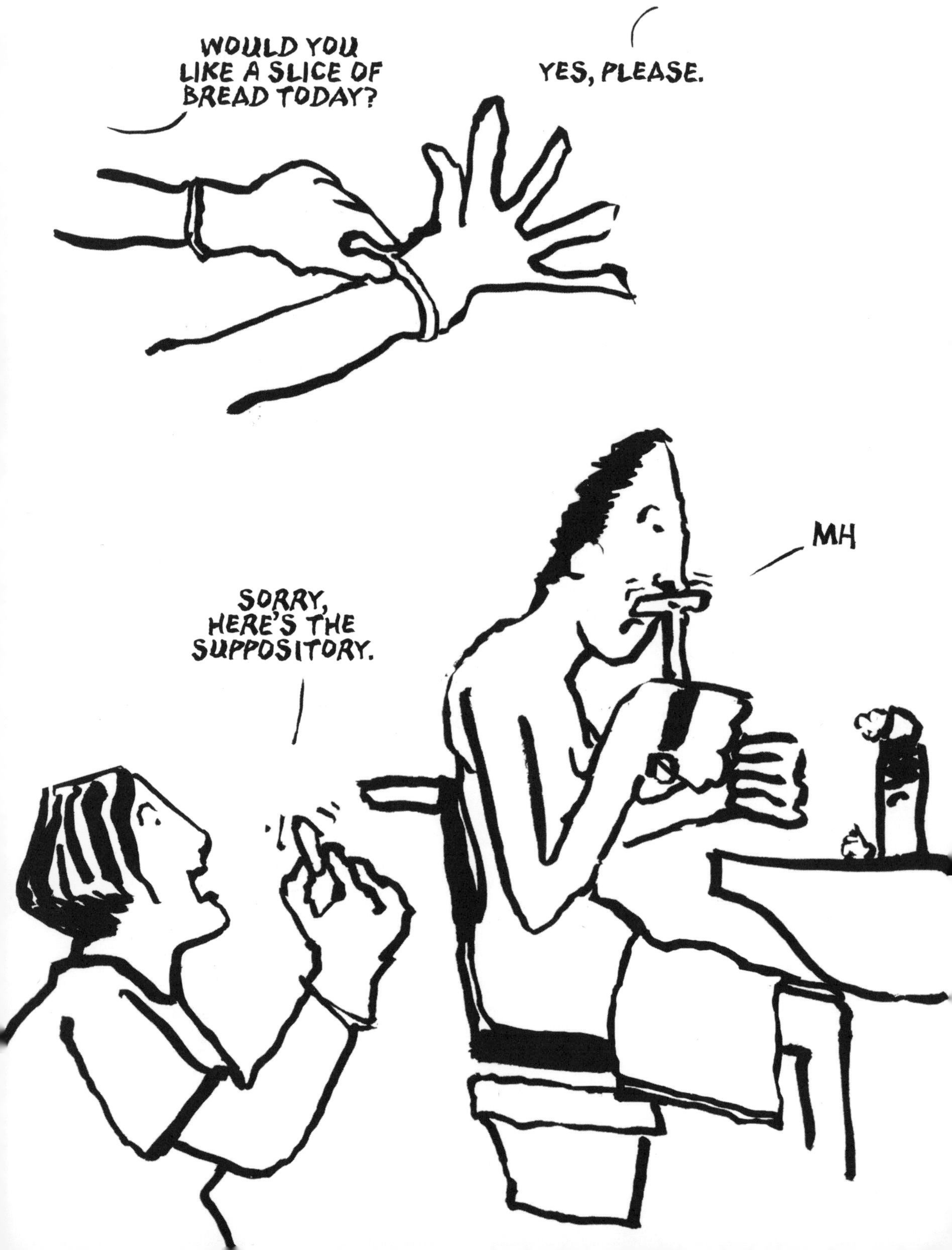
WOULD YOU LIKE A SLICE OF BREAD TODAY?
YES, PLEASE.
MH
SORRY, HERE'S THE SUPPOSITORY.

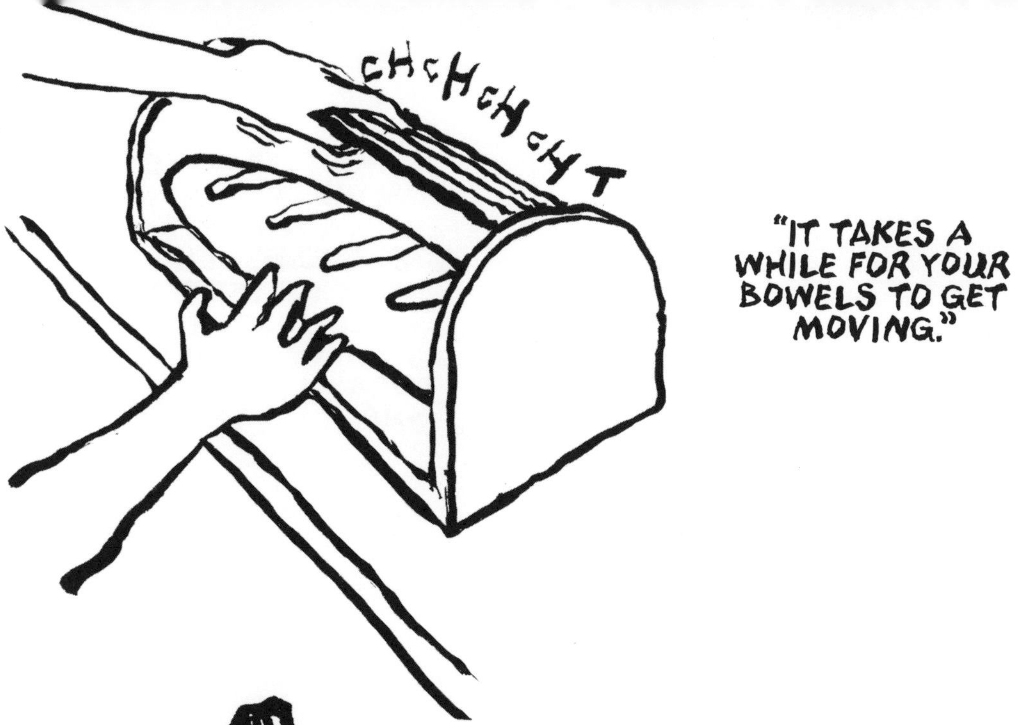
CHCHCHCHCHT
"IT TAKES A WHILE FOR YOUR BOWELS TO GET MOVING."

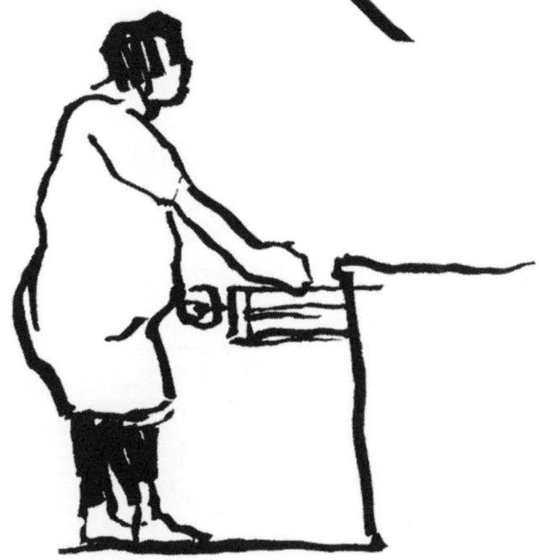

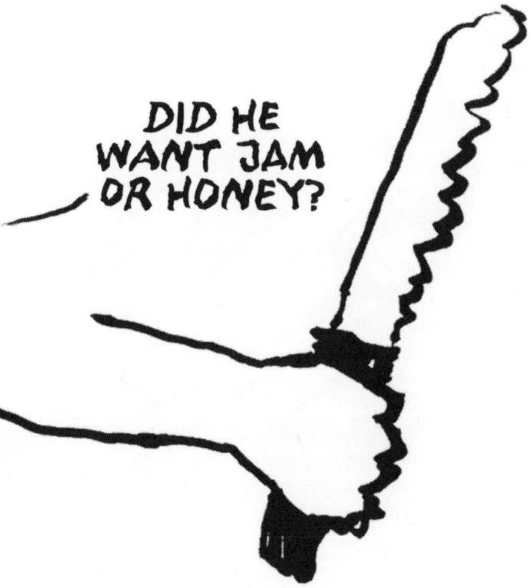
DID HE WANT JAM OR HONEY?

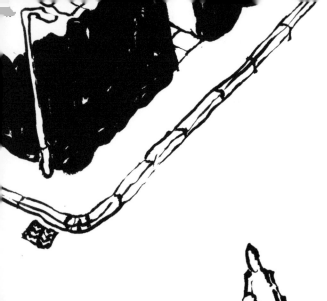

"WHEN WE WERE KIDS, WE EVEN WON A FEW SWIM MEETS AT OUR LOCAL CLUB. I WAS MORE OF A LONG-DISTANCE SWIMMER, WHILE LUCAS LOVED THE SHORTER RACES."

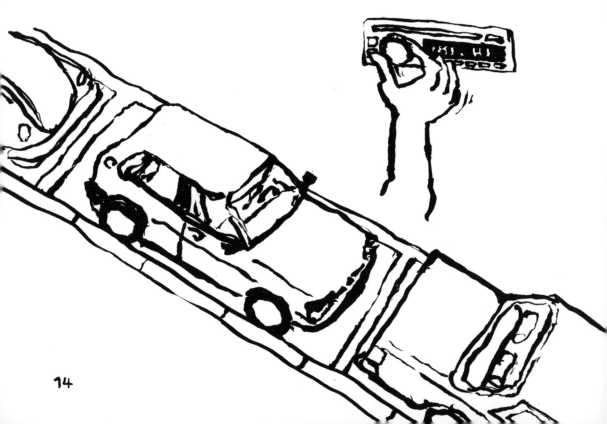

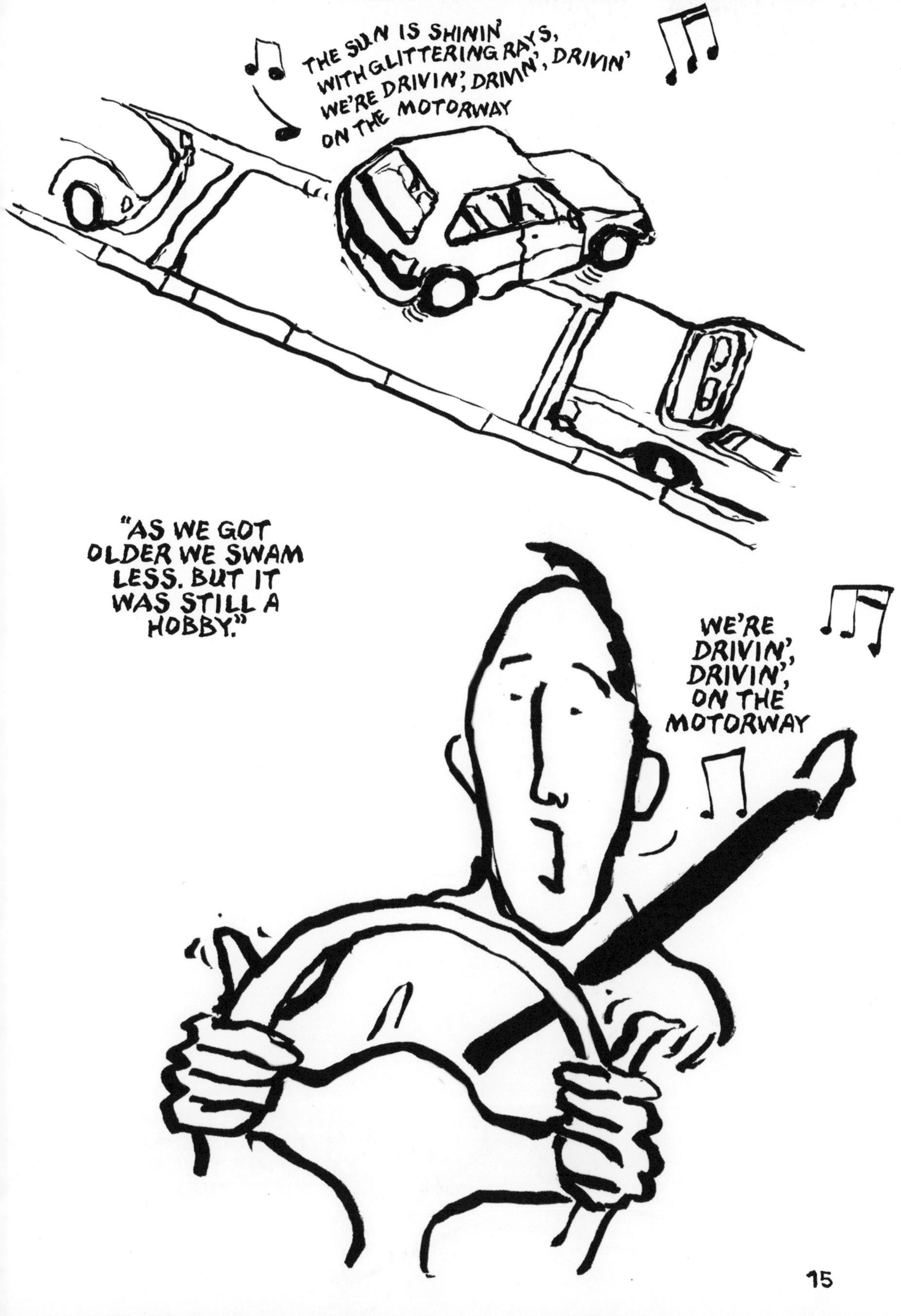
THE SUN IS SHININ' WITH GLITTERING RAYS, WE'RE DRIVIN', DRIVIN', DRIVIN' ON THE MOTORWAY
"AS WE GOT OLDER WE SWAM LESS. BUT IT WAS STILL A HOBBY."
WE'RE DRIVIN', DRIVIN', ON THE MOTORWAY

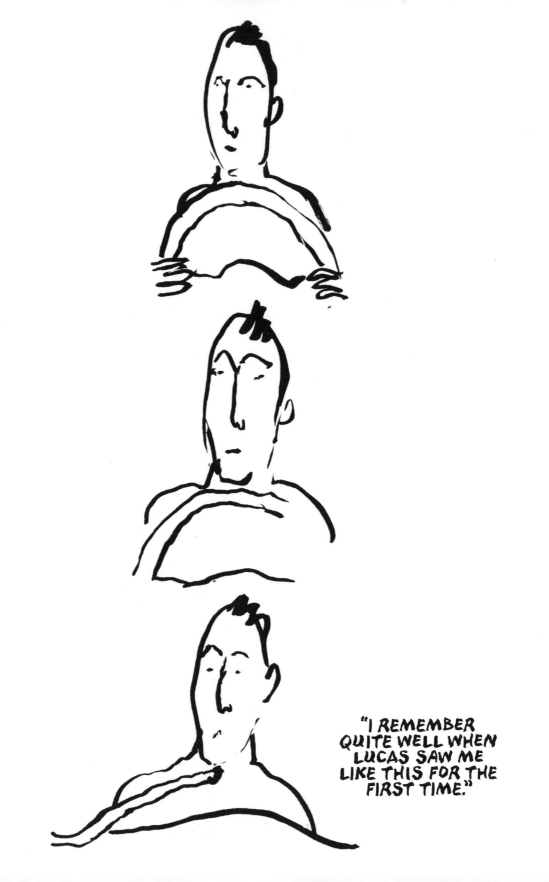

"I REMEMBER
QUITE WELL WHEN
LUCAS SAW ME
LIKE THIS FOR THE
FIRST TIME."

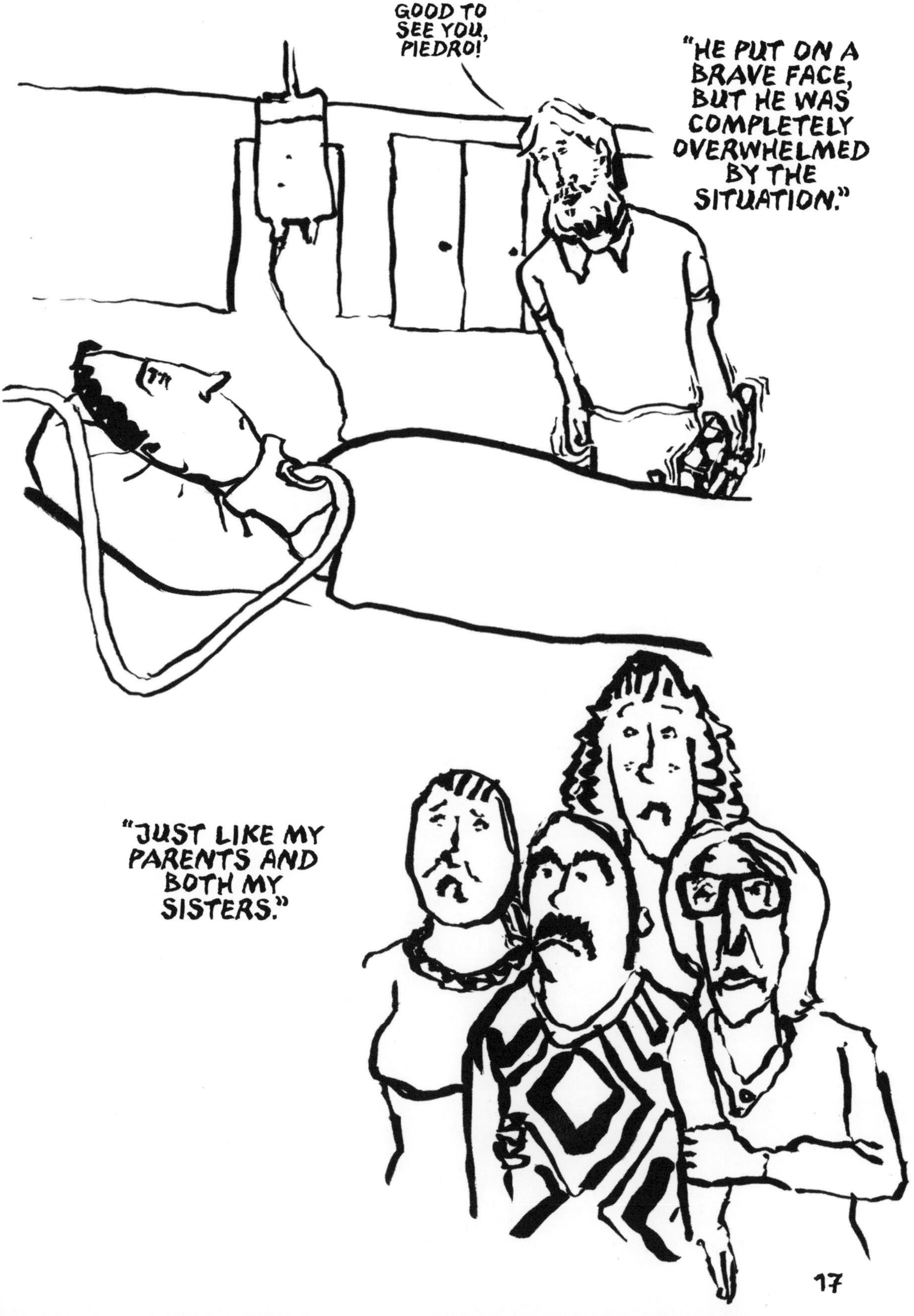
GOOD TO SEE YOU, PIEDRO!
"HE PUT ON A BRAVE FACE, BUT HE WAS COMPLETELY OVERWHELMED BY THE SITUATION."
"JUST LIKE MY PARENTS AND BOTH MY SISTERS."

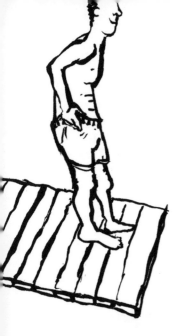

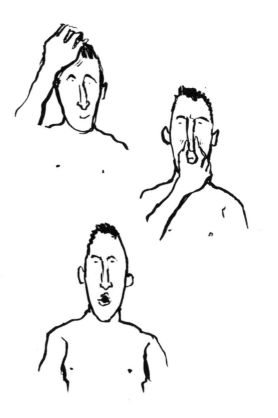

"IT ALL HAPPENED
REALLY FAST. BUT
TO ME, IT FELT LIKE
AN ETERNITY."

"I STILL REMEMBER
DIVING INTO THE WATER.
AND THEN I HIT MY
HEAD ON SOMETHING
HARD."

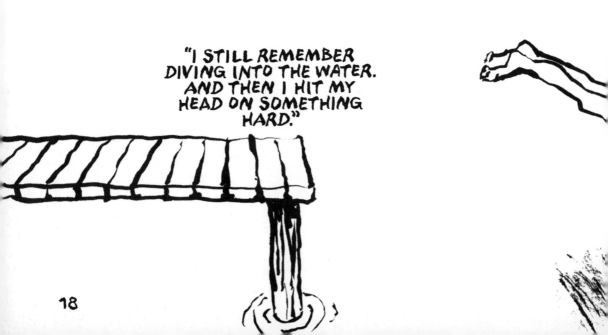

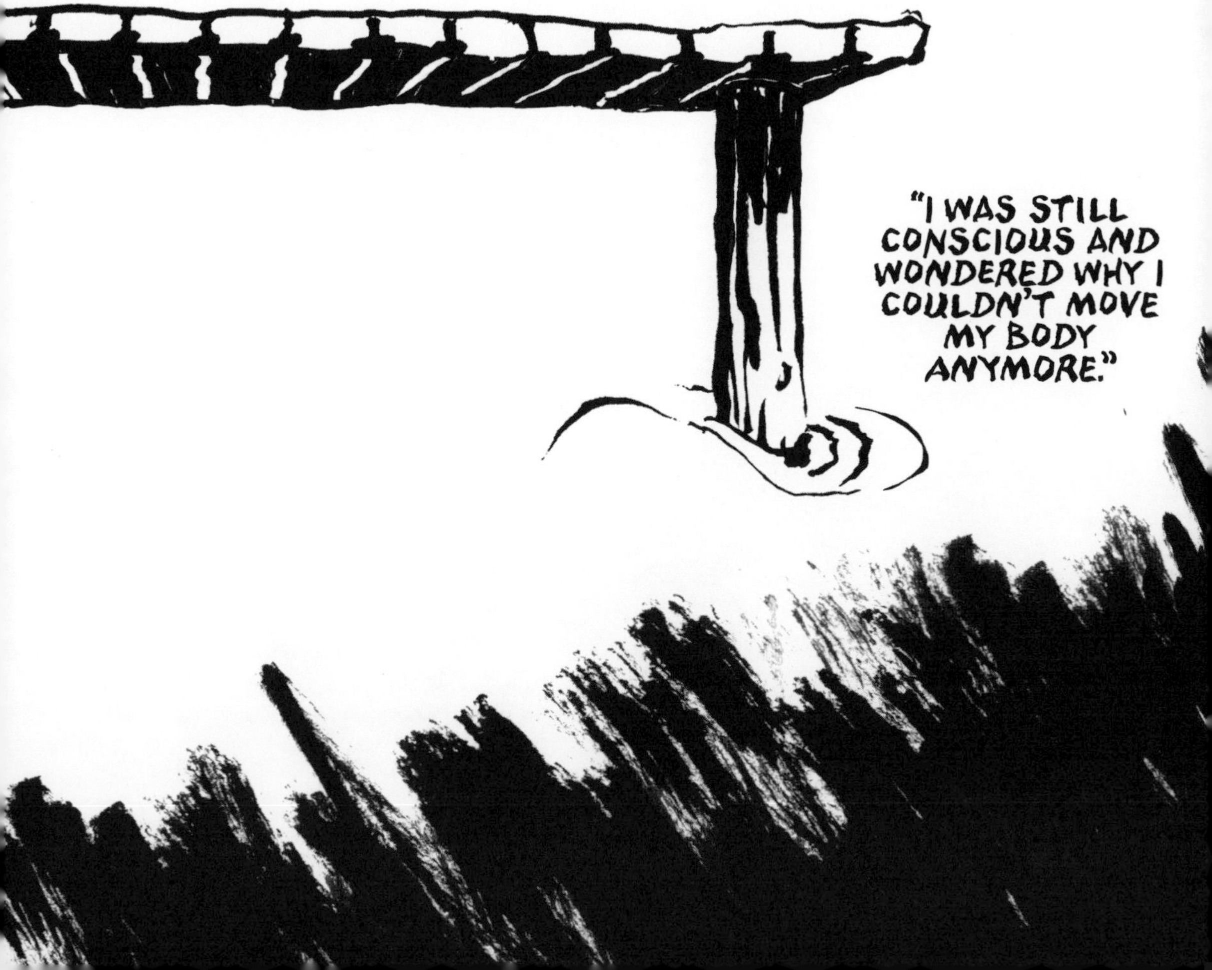
"I WAS STILL CONSCIOUS AND WONDERED WHY I COULDN'T MOVE MY BODY ANYMORE."

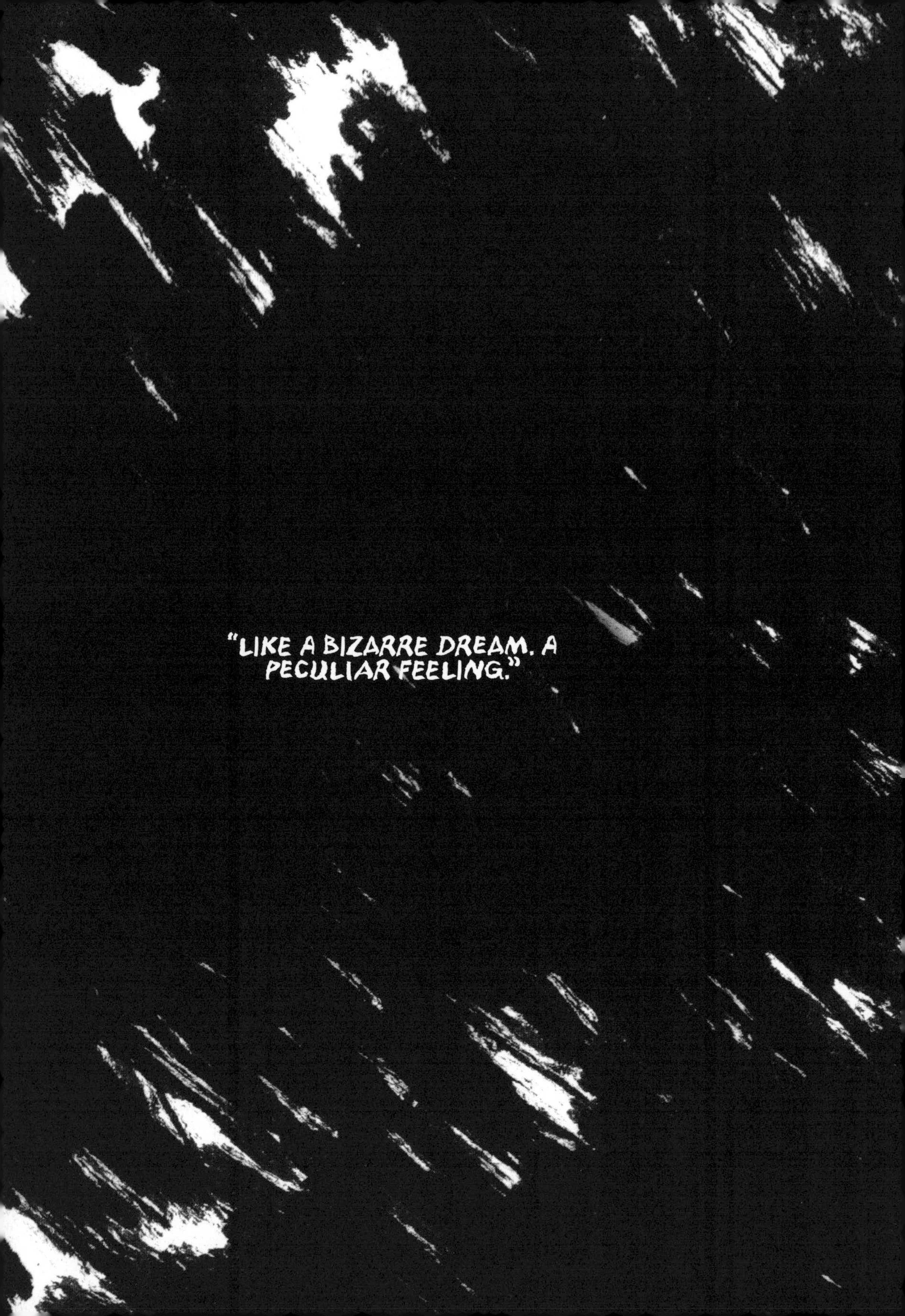
"LIKE A BIZARRE DREAM. A PECULIAR FEELING."

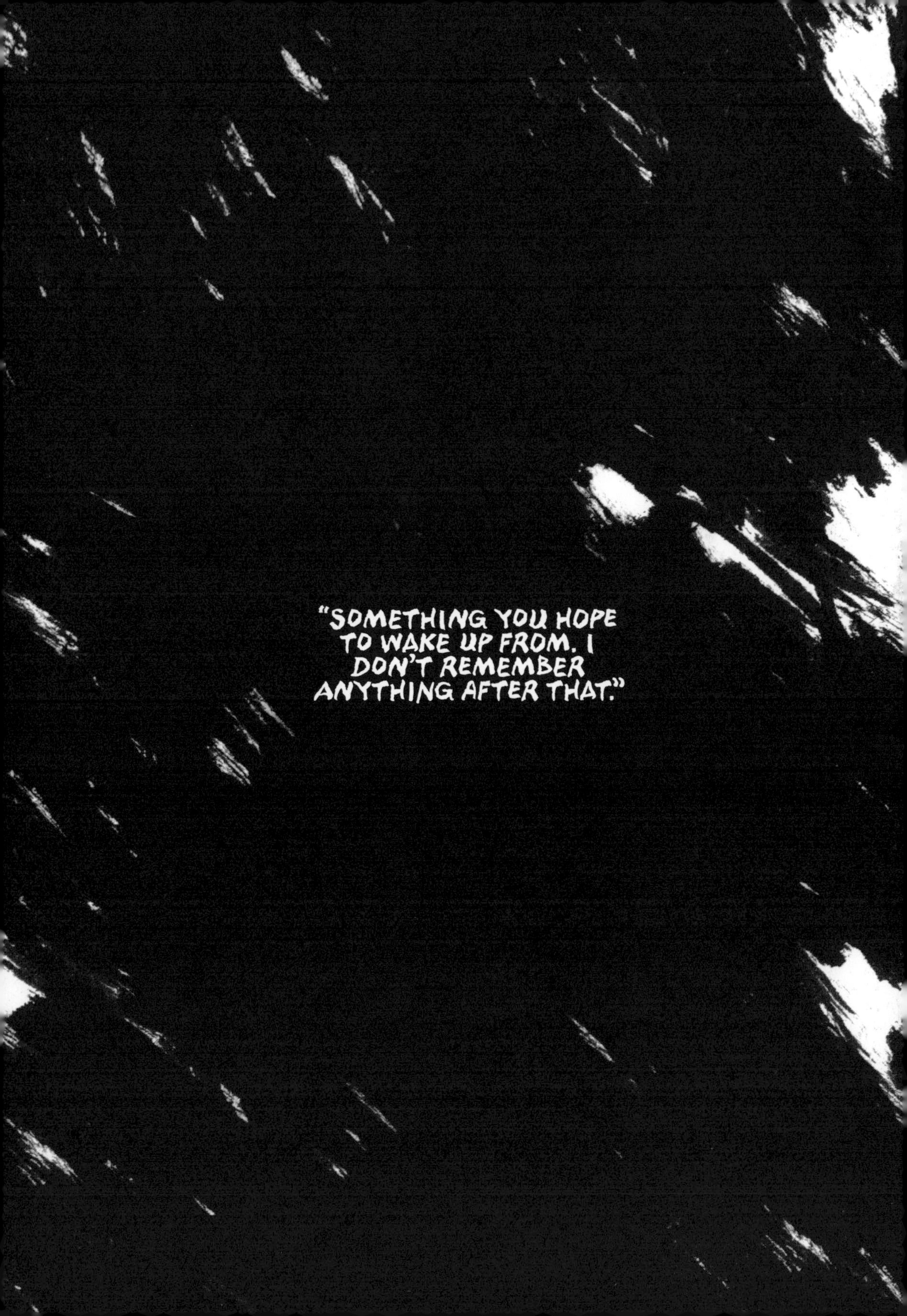
"SOMETHING YOU HOPE TO WAKE UP FROM. I DON'T REMEMBER ANYTHING AFTER THAT."

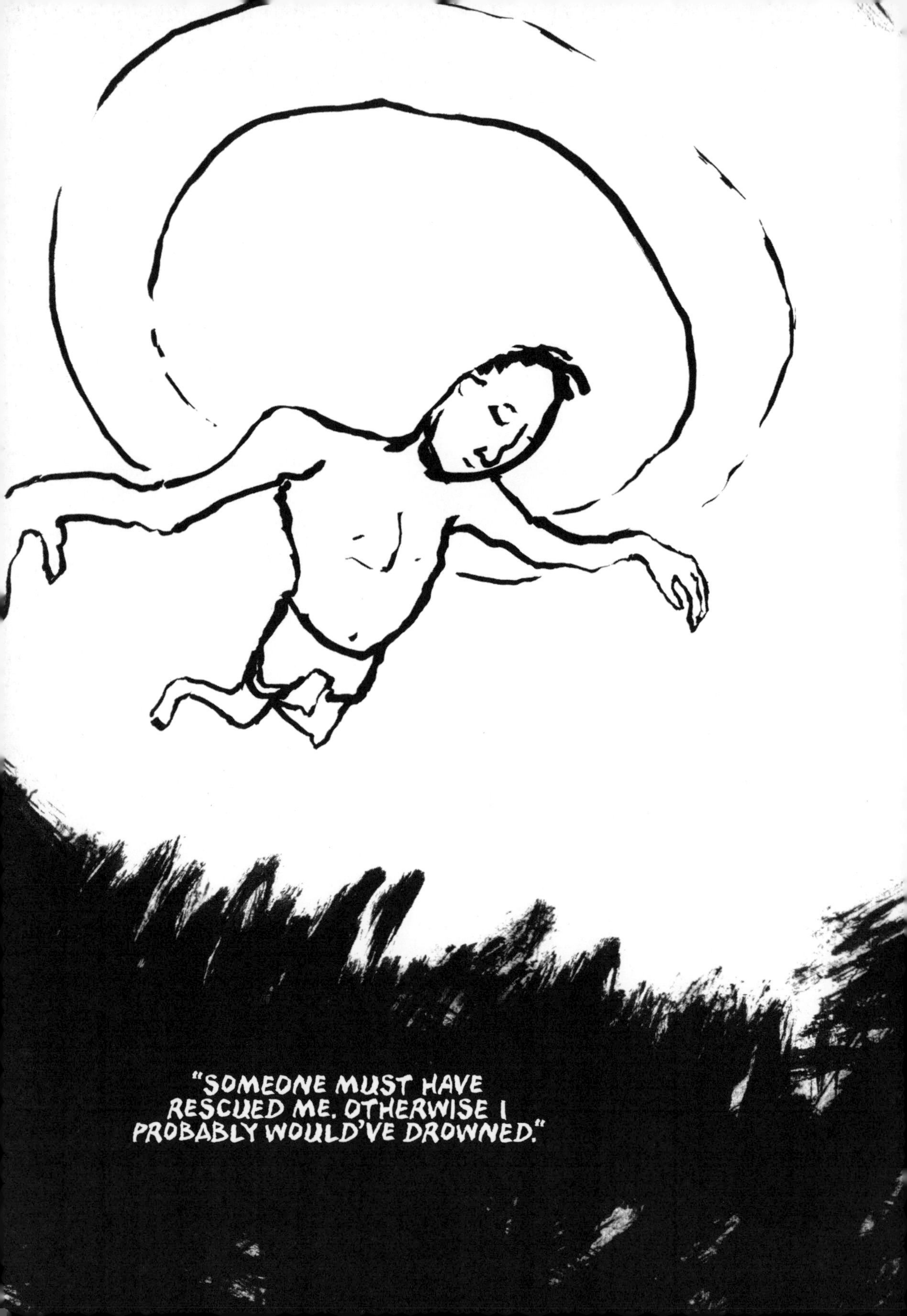
"SOMEONE MUST HAVE
RESCUED ME. OTHERWISE I
PROBABLY WOULD'VE DROWNED."

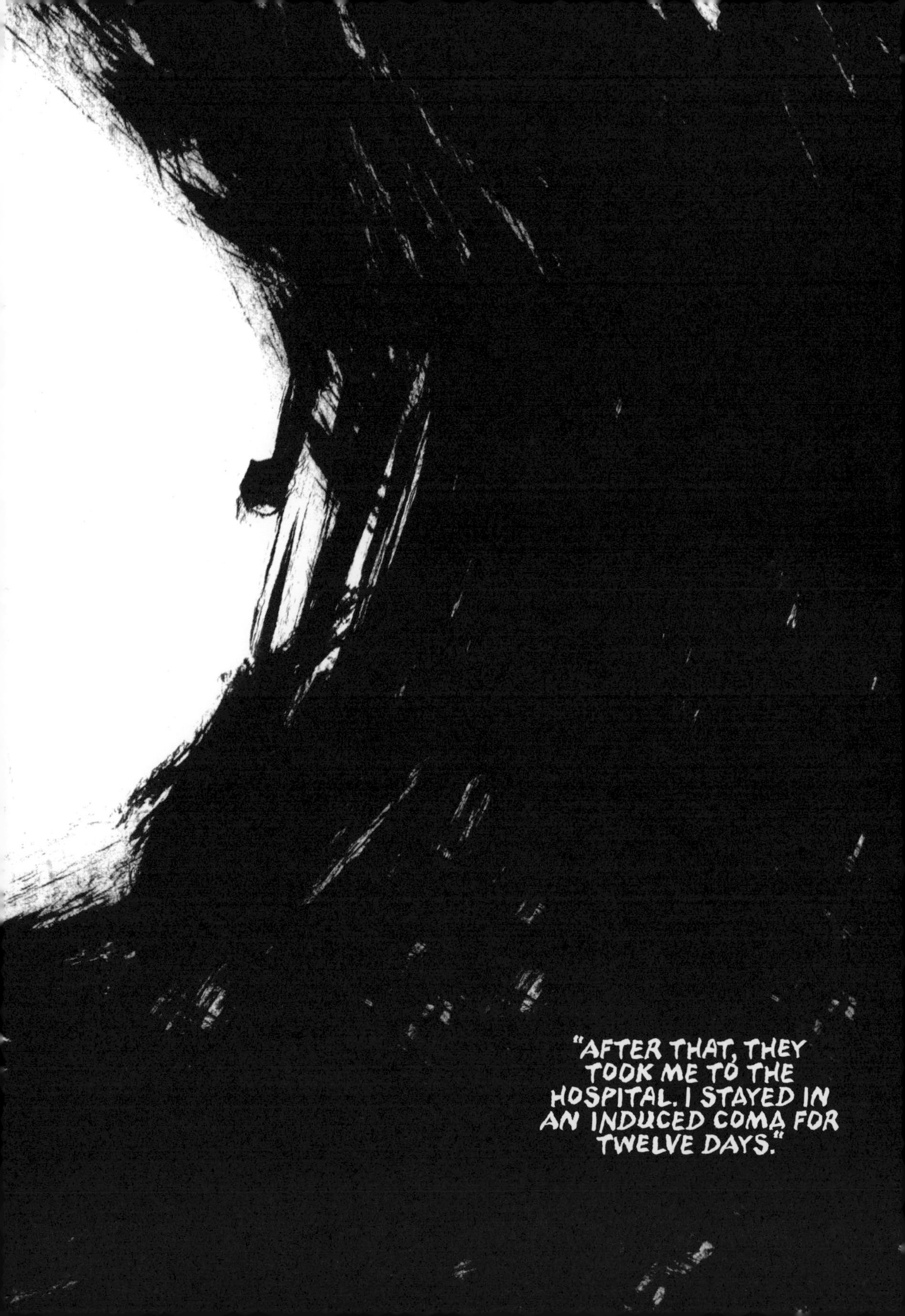
"AFTER THAT, THEY TOOK ME TO THE HOSPITAL. I STAYED IN AN INDUCED COMA FOR TWELVE DAYS."

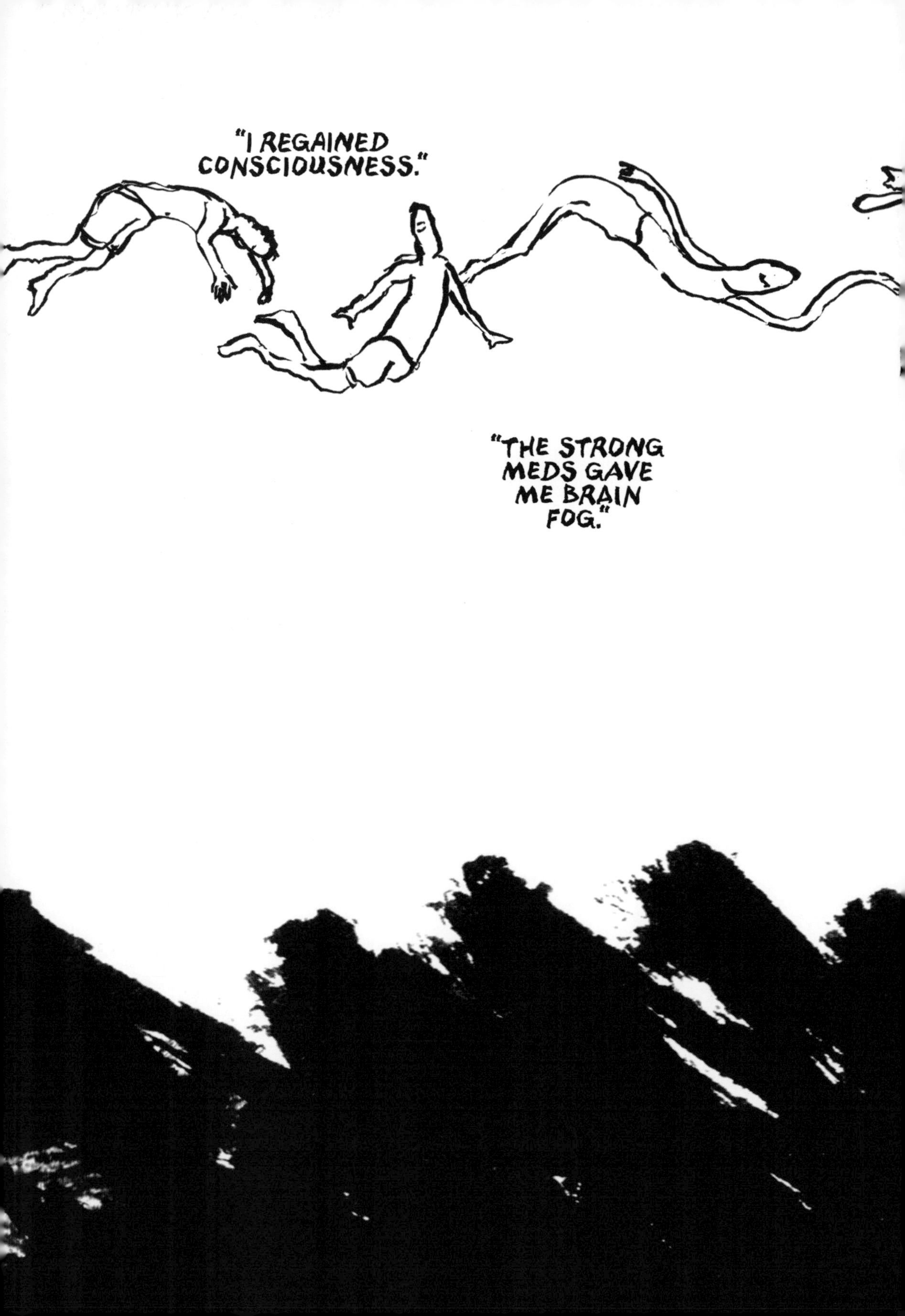
"I REGAINED CONSCIOUSNESS."
"THE STRONG MEDS GAVE ME BRAIN FOG."

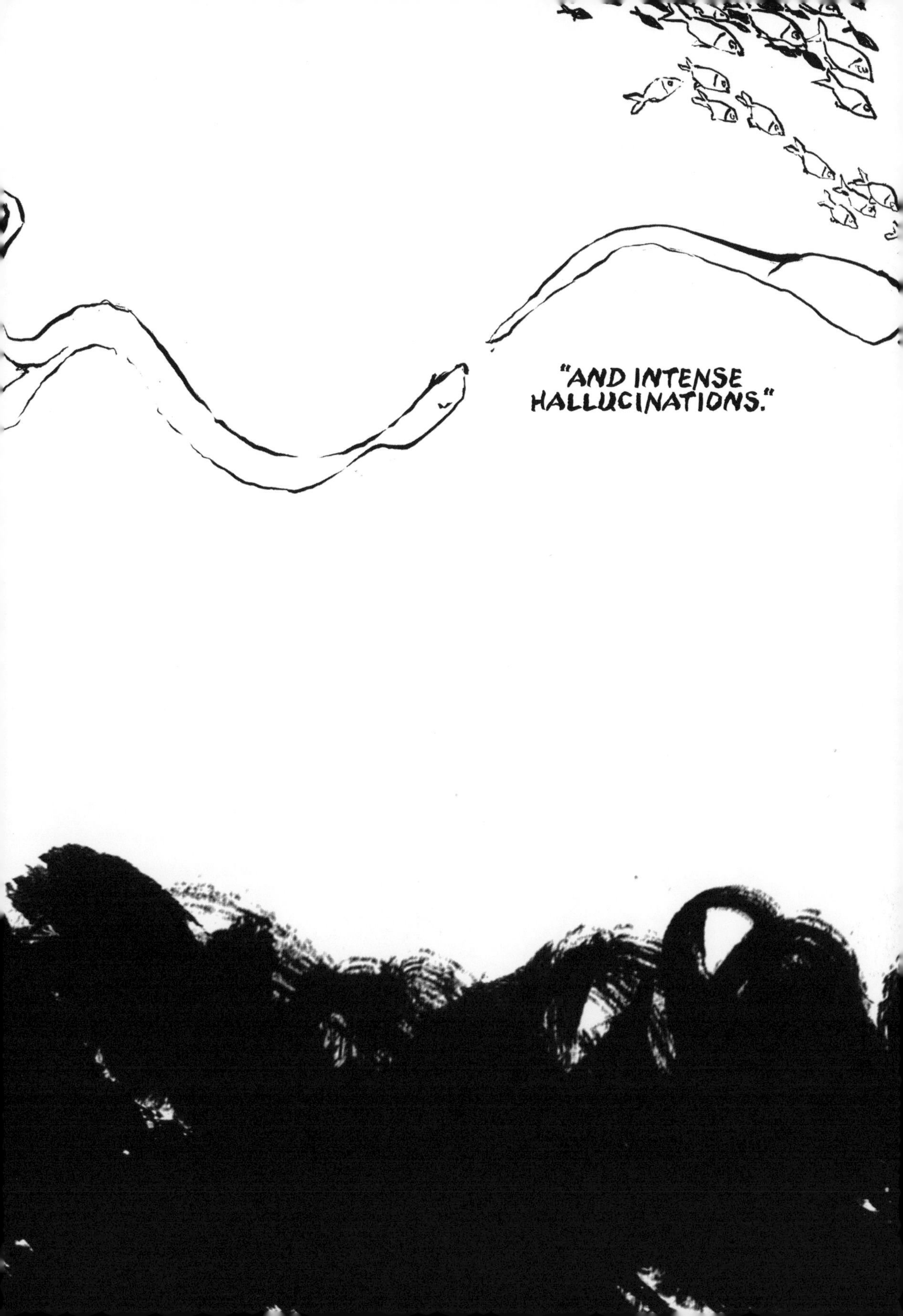
"AND INTENSE HALLUCINATIONS."

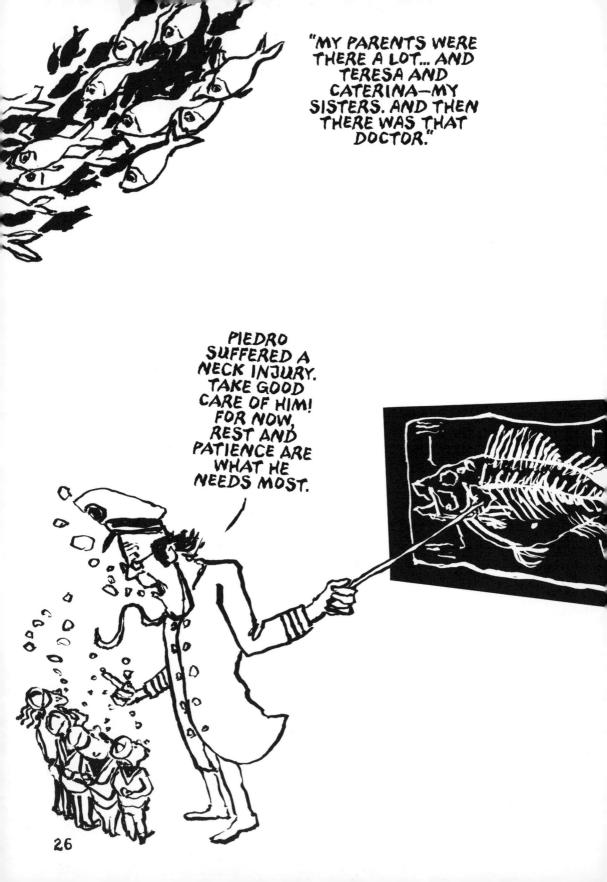

"MY PARENTS WERE THERE A LOT... AND TERESA AND CATERINA—MY SISTERS. AND THEN THERE WAS THAT DOCTOR."

PIEDRO SUFFERED A NECK INJURY. TAKE GOOD CARE OF HIM! FOR NOW, REST AND PATIENCE ARE WHAT HE NEEDS MOST.

26

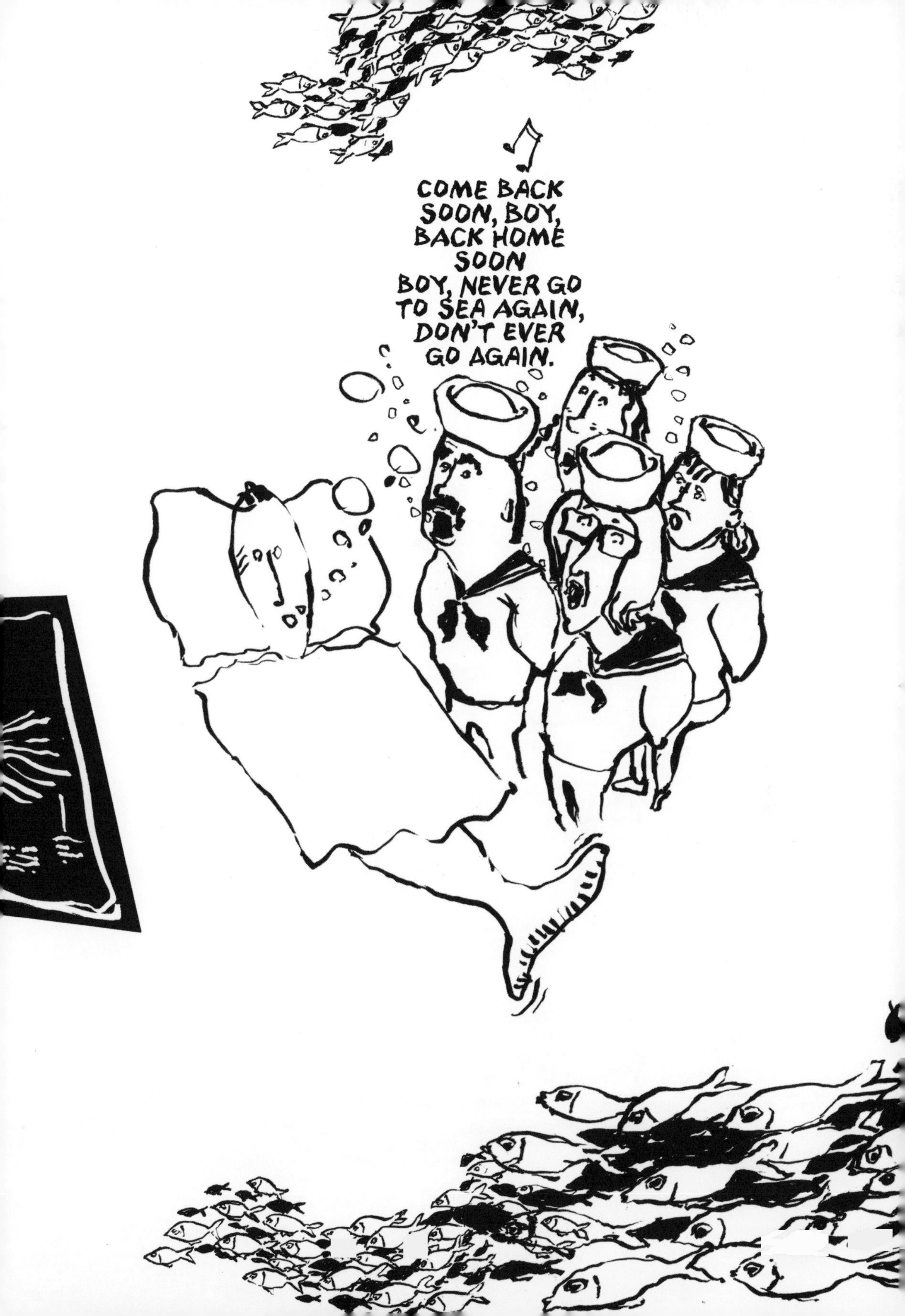
COME BACK SOON, BOY, BACK HOME SOON BOY, NEVER GO TO SEA AGAIN, DON'T EVER GO AGAIN.

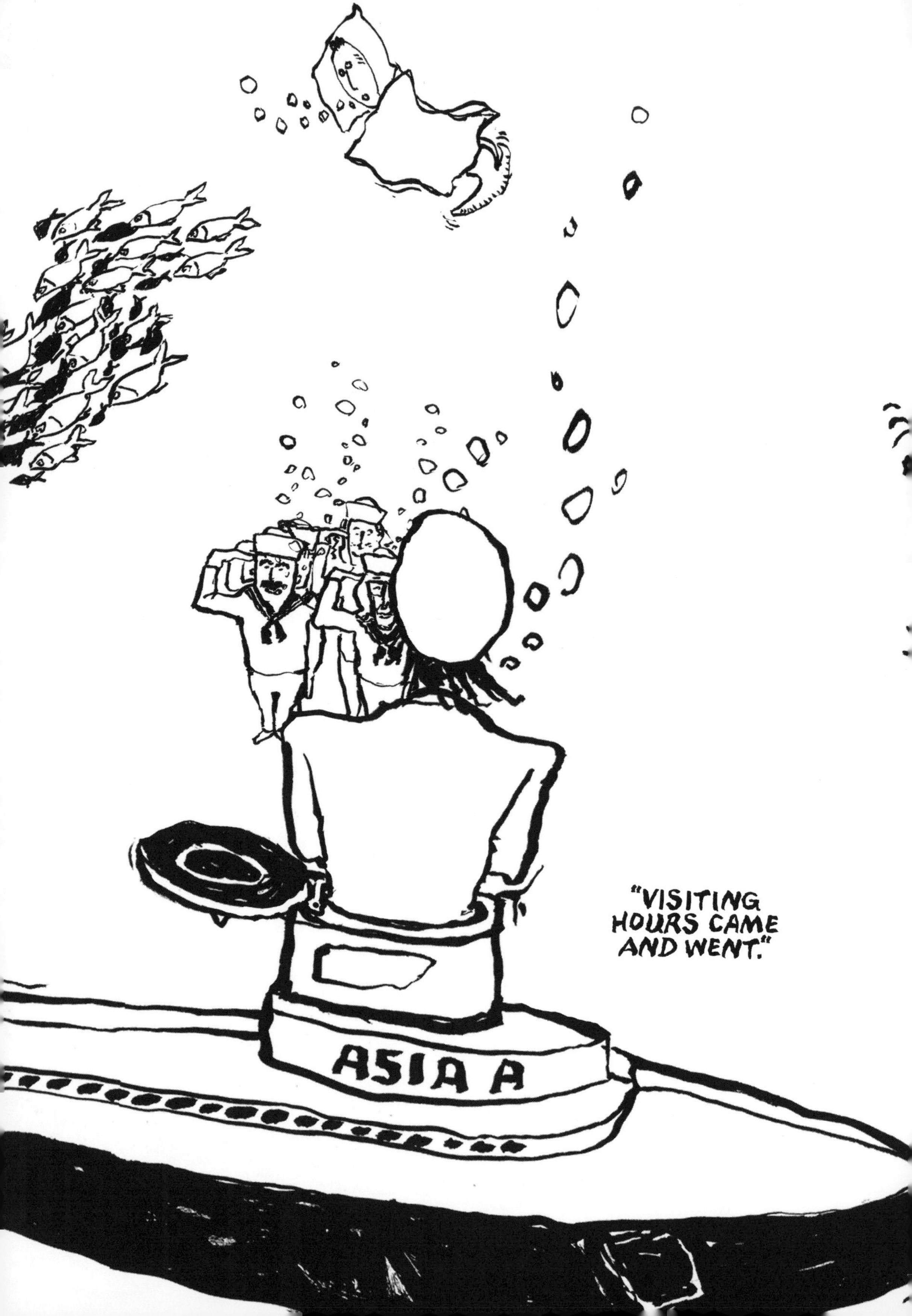
"VISITING
HOURS CAME
AND WENT."
ASIA A

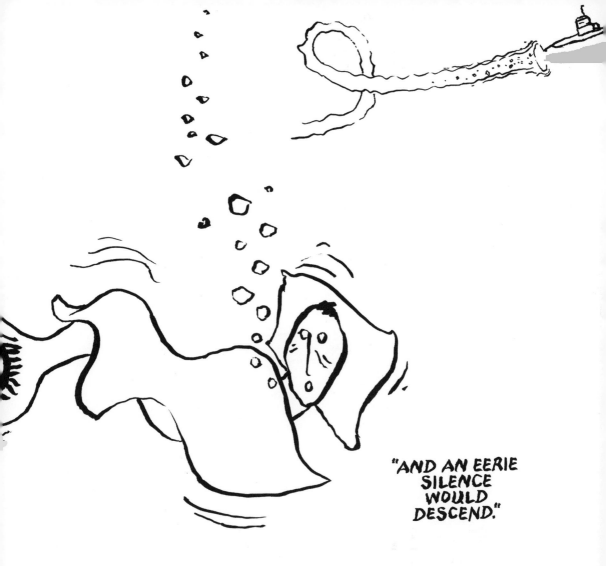

"AND AN EERIE
SILENCE
WOULD
DESCEND."

"I FLOATED,
LONELY, IN THE
OCEAN."

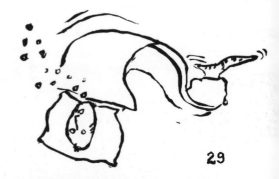

"NOWADAYS, I APPRECIATE THESE RARE MOMENTS OF QUIET A LOT MORE."

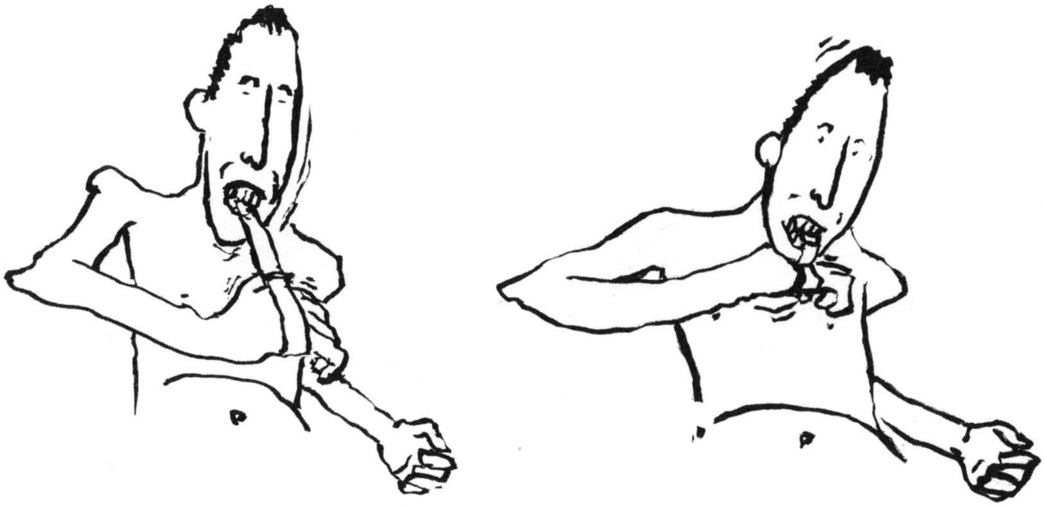

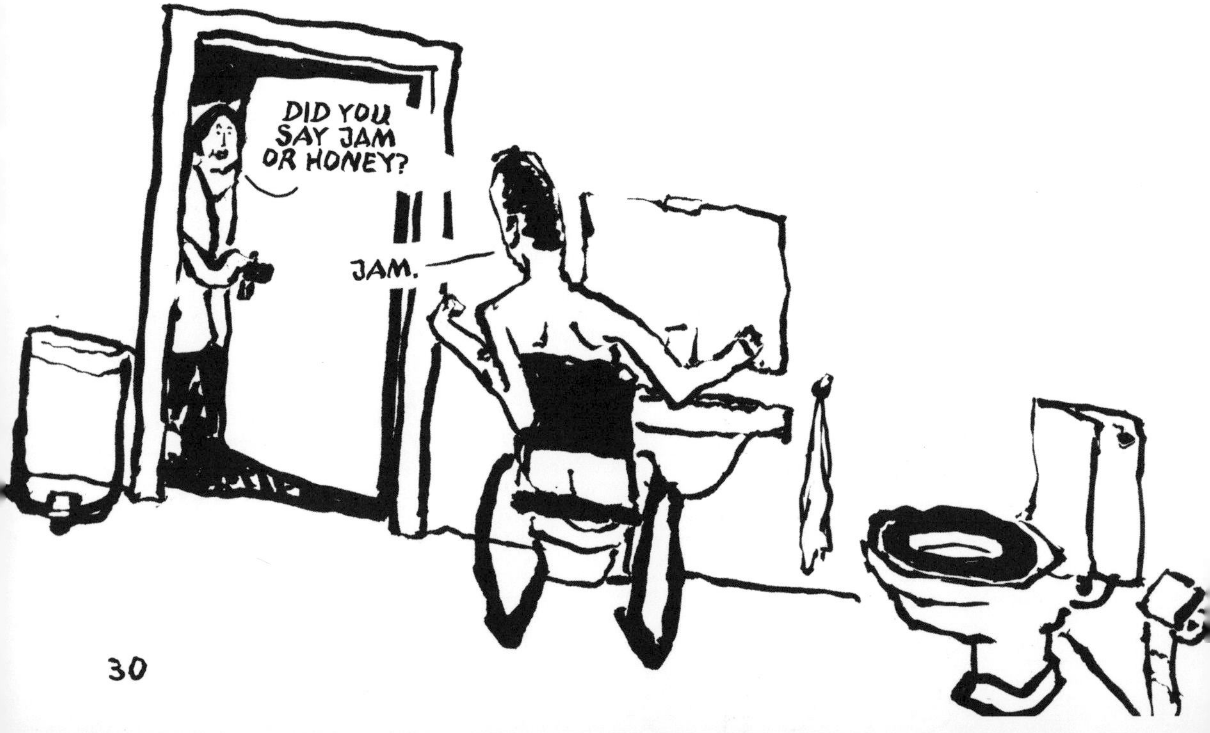
DID YOU SAY JAM OR HONEY?
JAM.

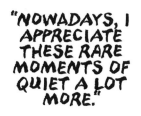

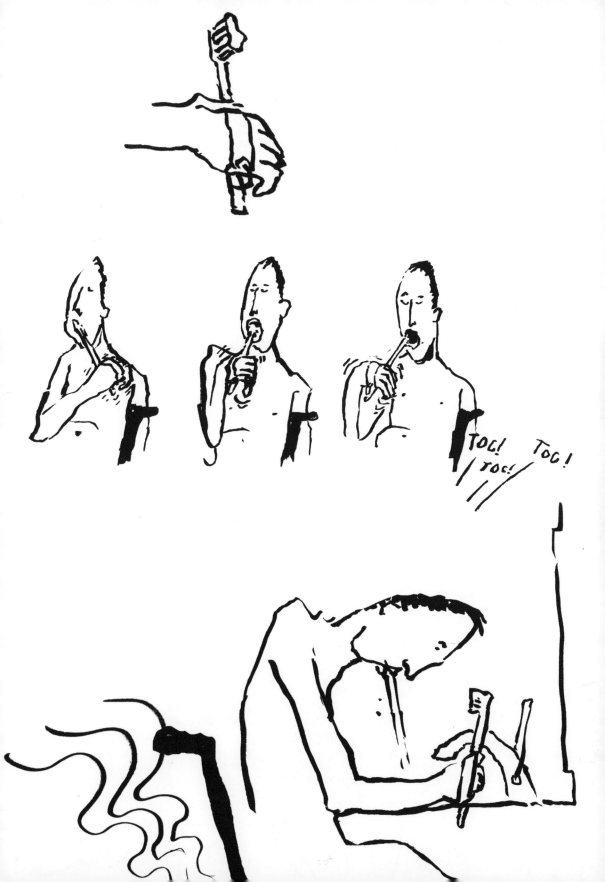

TOC! TOC!
TOC!

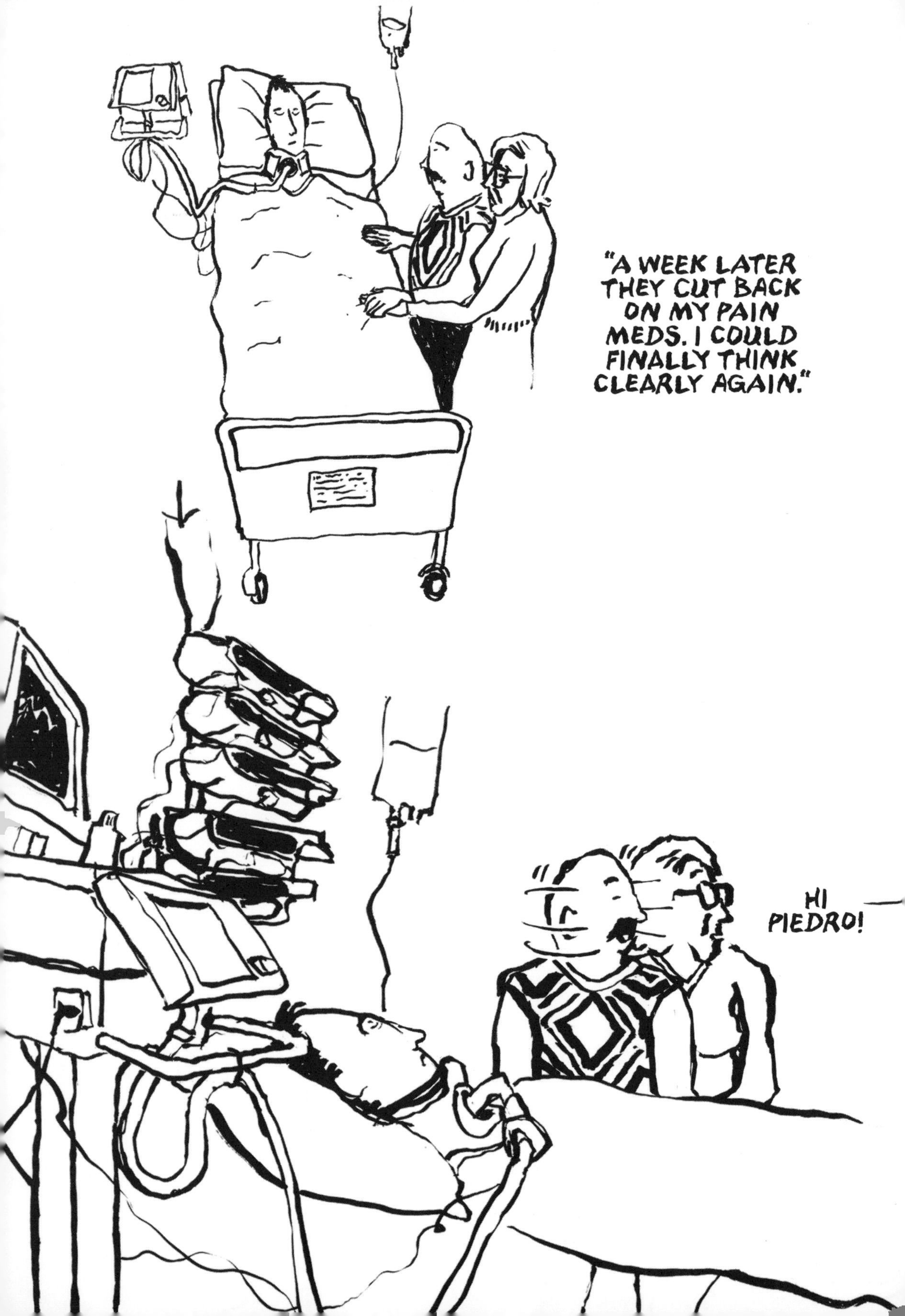
"A WEEK LATER THEY CUT BACK ON MY PAIN MEDS. I COULD FINALLY THINK CLEARLY AGAIN."
HI PIEDRO!

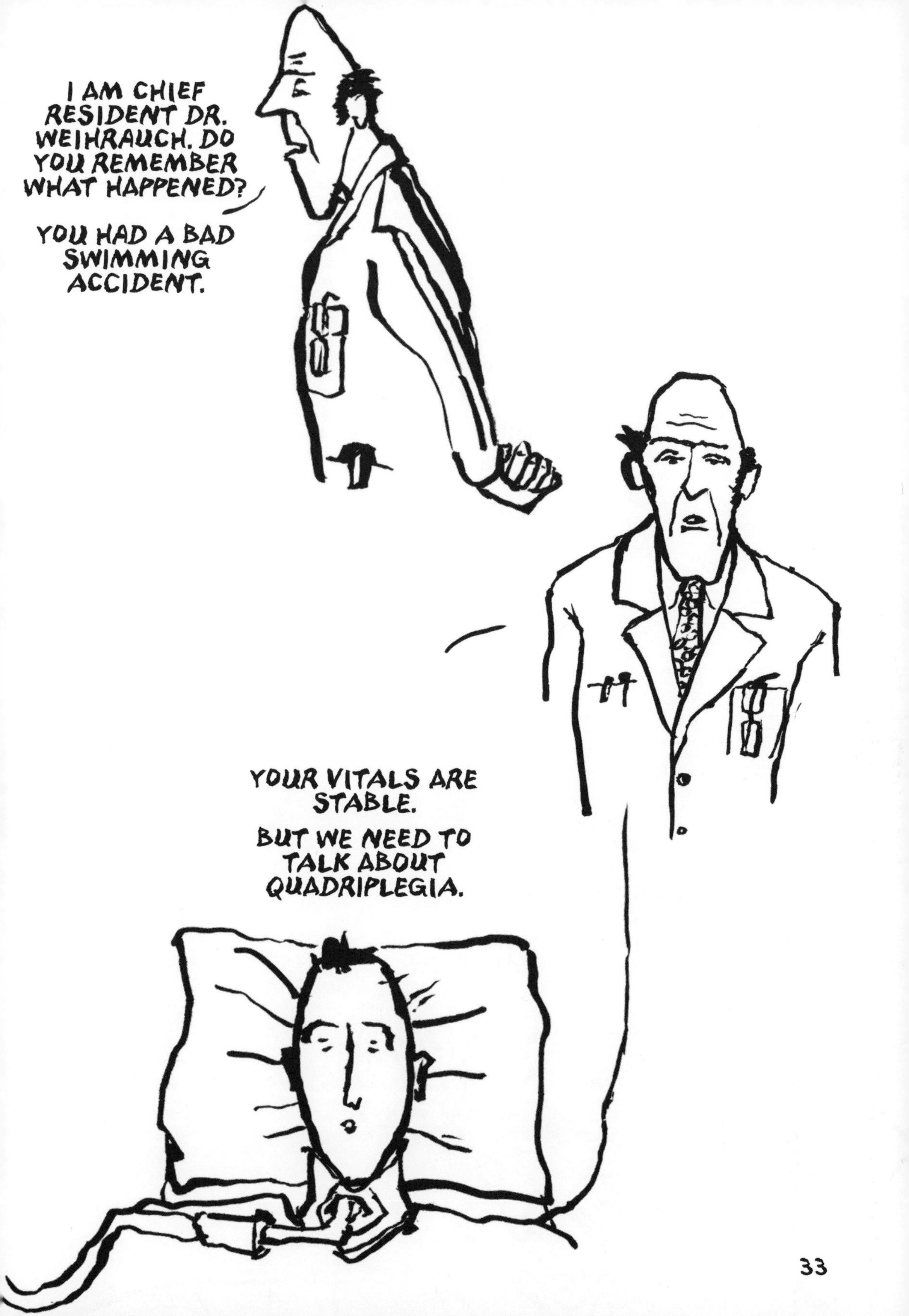
I AM CHIEF RESIDENT DR. WEIHRAUCH. DO YOU REMEMBER WHAT HAPPENED?
YOU HAD A BAD SWIMMING ACCIDENT.
YOUR VITALS ARE STABLE.
BUT WE NEED TO TALK ABOUT QUADRIPLEGIA.

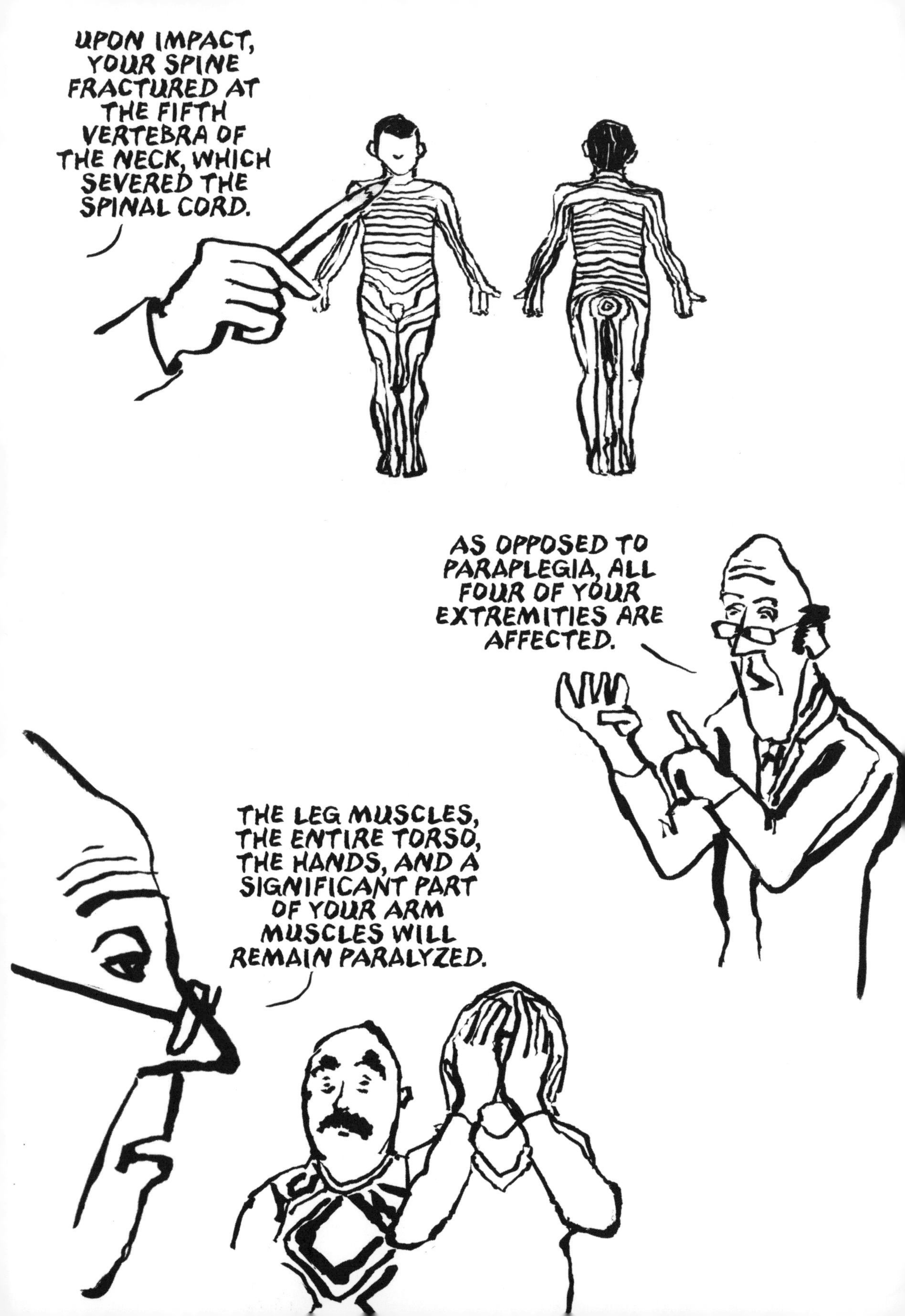
UPON IMPACT, YOUR SPINE FRACTURED AT THE FIFTH VERTEBRA OF THE NECK, WHICH SEVERED THE SPINAL CORD.
AS OPPOSED TO PARAPLEGIA, ALL FOUR OF YOUR EXTREMITIES ARE AFFECTED.
THE LEG MUSCLES, THE ENTIRE TORSO, THE HANDS, AND A SIGNIFICANT PART OF YOUR ARM MUSCLES WILL REMAIN PARALYZED.

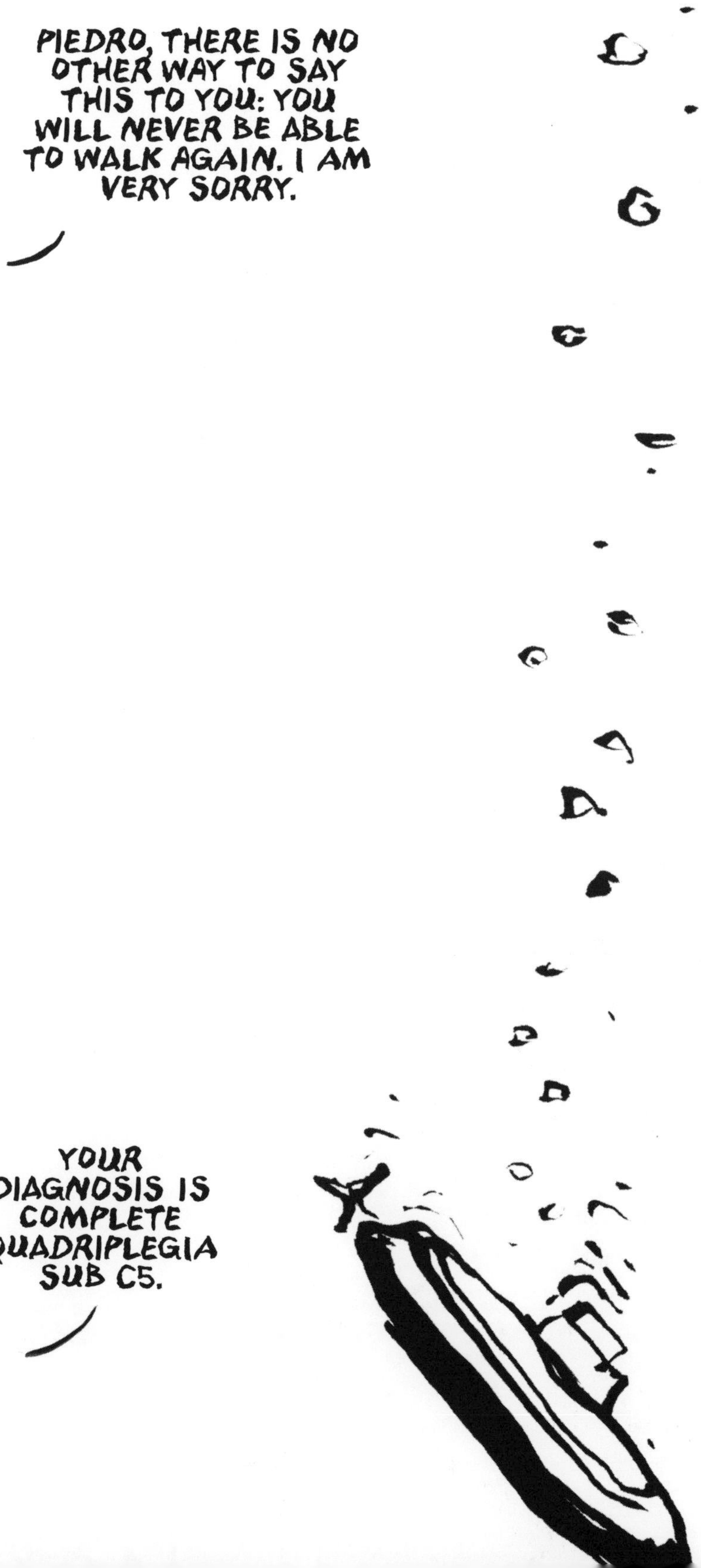
PIEDRO, THERE IS NO OTHER WAY TO SAY THIS TO YOU: YOU WILL NEVER BE ABLE TO WALK AGAIN. I AM VERY SORRY.
YOUR DIAGNOSIS IS COMPLETE QUADRIPLEGIA SUB C5.

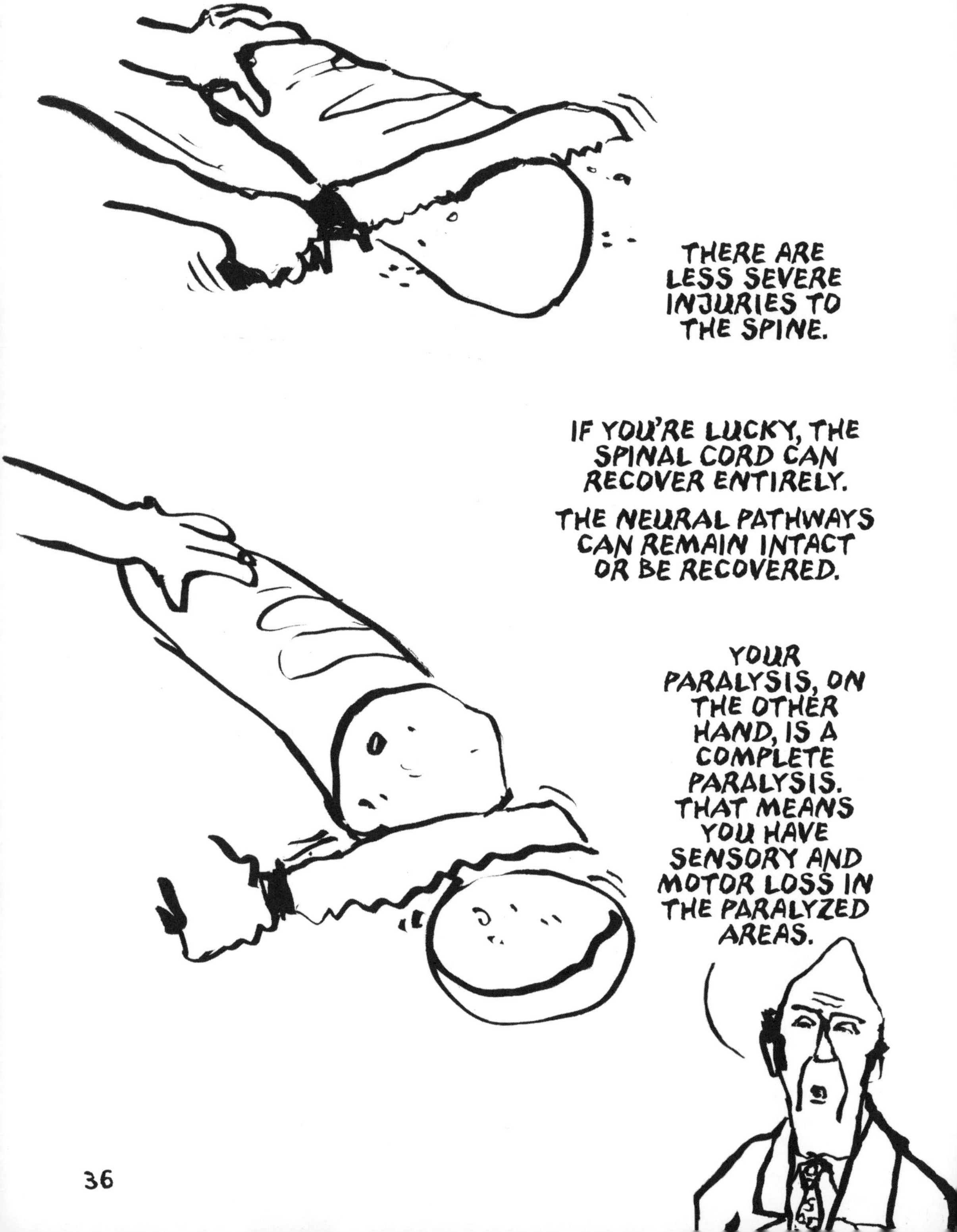
THERE ARE LESS SEVERE INJURIES TO THE SPINE.
IF YOU'RE LUCKY, THE SPINAL CORD CAN RECOVER ENTIRELY.
THE NEURAL PATHWAYS CAN REMAIN INTACT OR BE RECOVERED.
YOUR PARALYSIS, ON THE OTHER HAND, IS A COMPLETE PARALYSIS. THAT MEANS YOU HAVE SENSORY AND MOTOR LOSS IN THE PARALYZED AREAS.

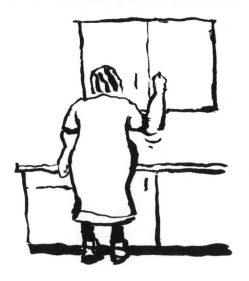

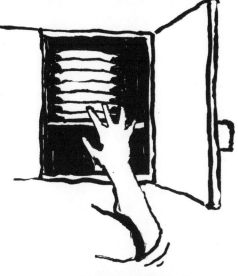

THE DAY AFTER YOUR ACCIDENT, WE PERFORMED EMERGENCY SURGERY TO STABILIZE YOUR SPINE.

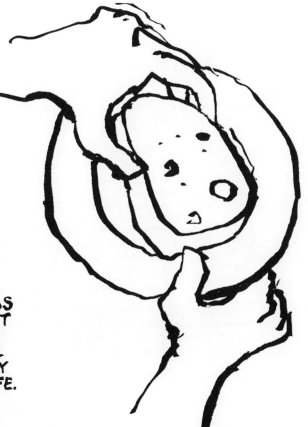

THE SURGERY WAS SUCCESSFUL. BUT THIS NEW CONDITION WILL FUNDAMENTALLY CHANGE YOUR LIFE.

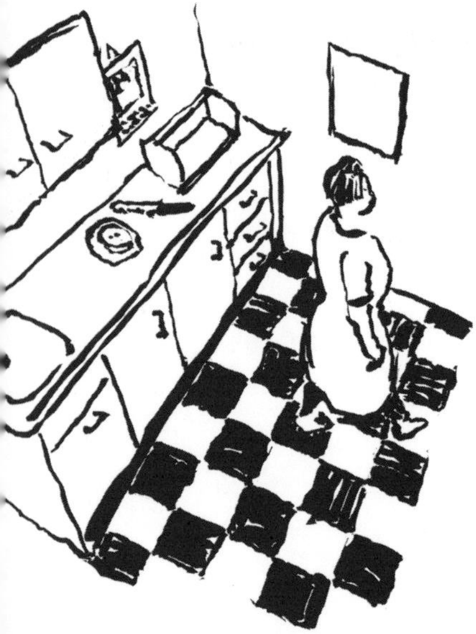

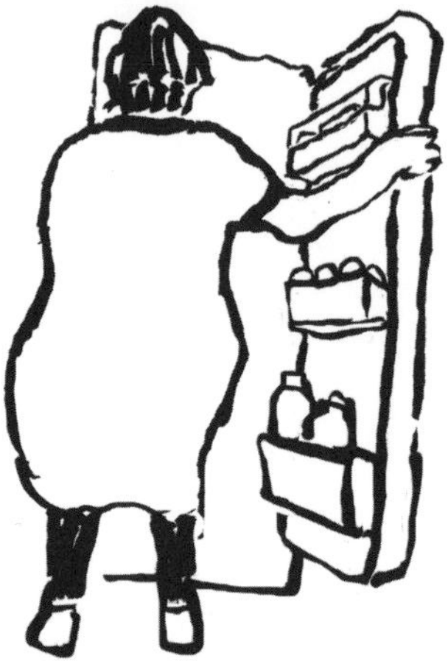

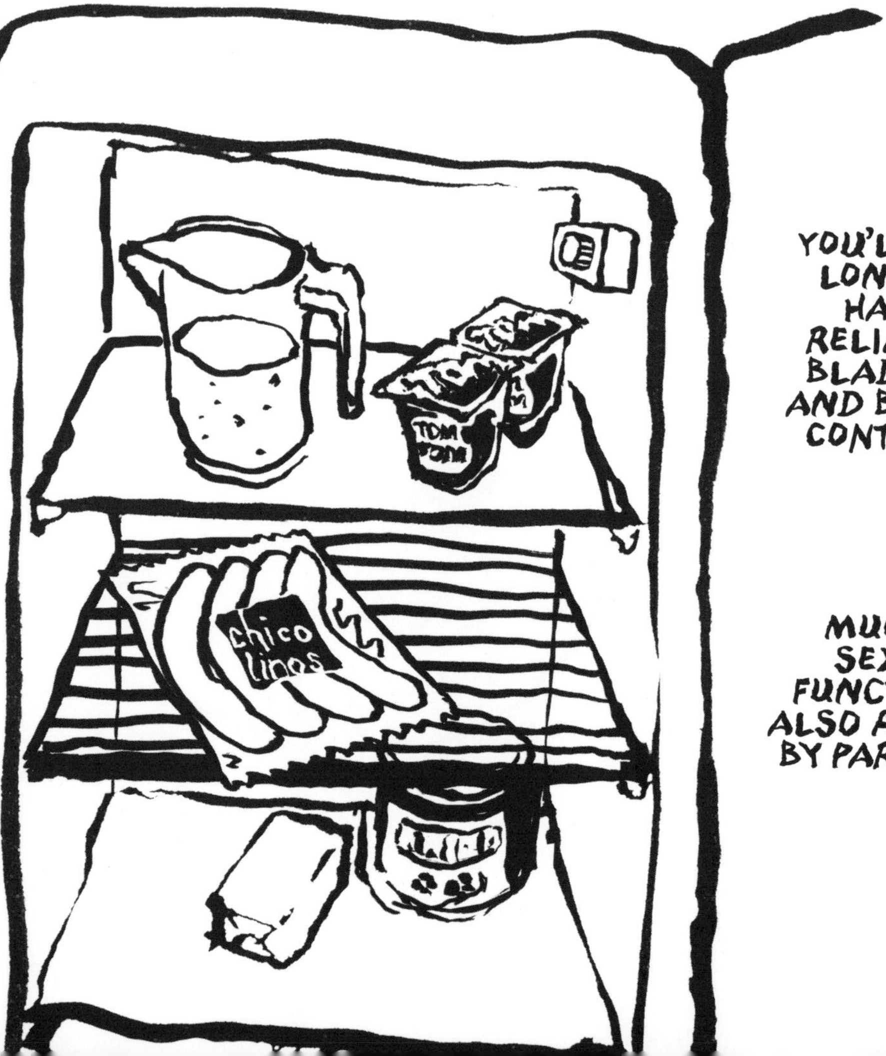

YOU'LL NO LONGER HAVE RELIABLE BLADDER AND BOWEL CONTROL.

MUCH OF SEXUAL FUNCTION IS ALSO AFFECTED BY PARALYSIS.

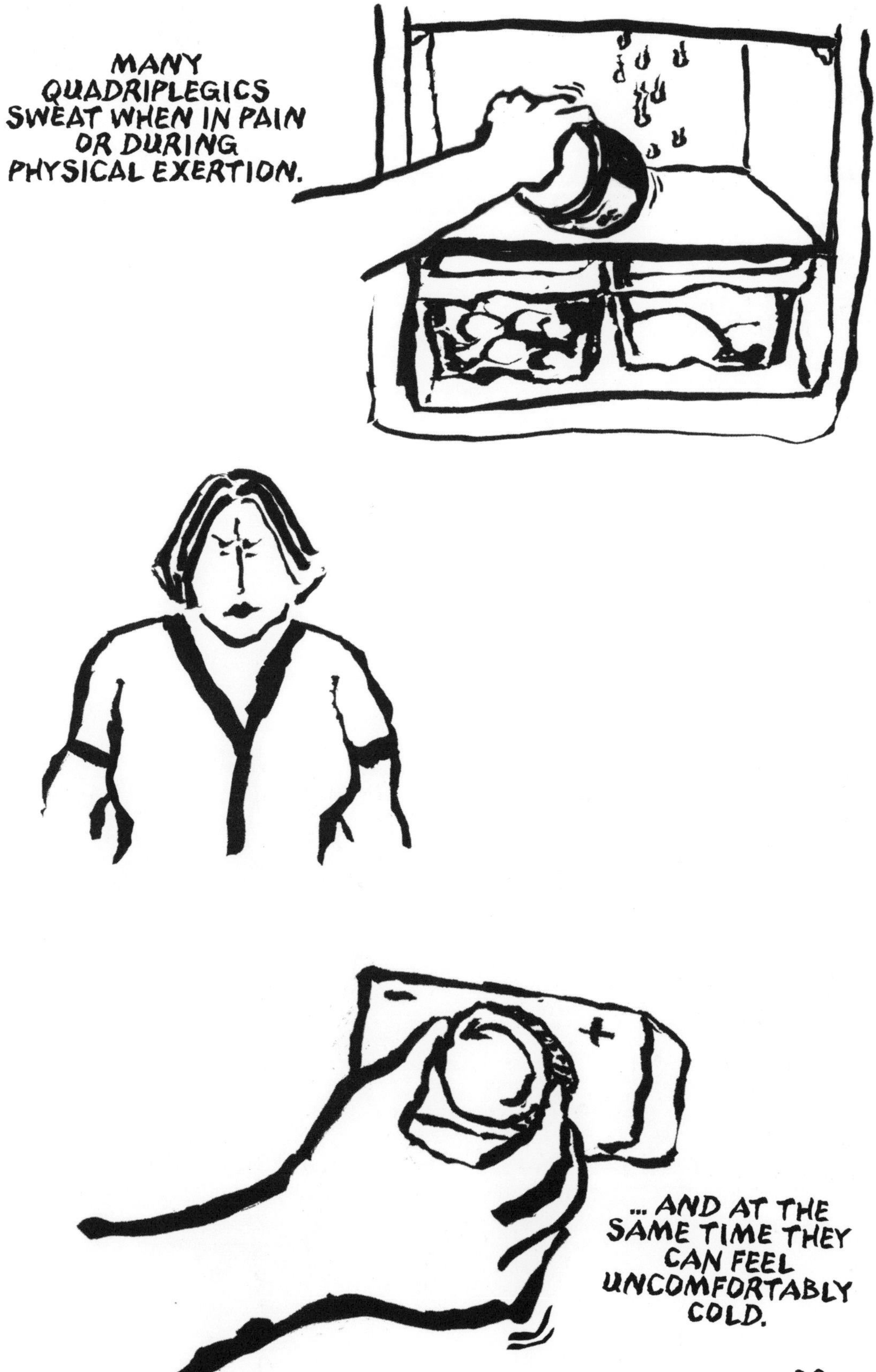
MANY QUADRIPLEGICS SWEAT WHEN IN PAIN OR DURING PHYSICAL EXERTION.
... AND AT THE SAME TIME THEY CAN FEEL UNCOMFORTABLY COLD.

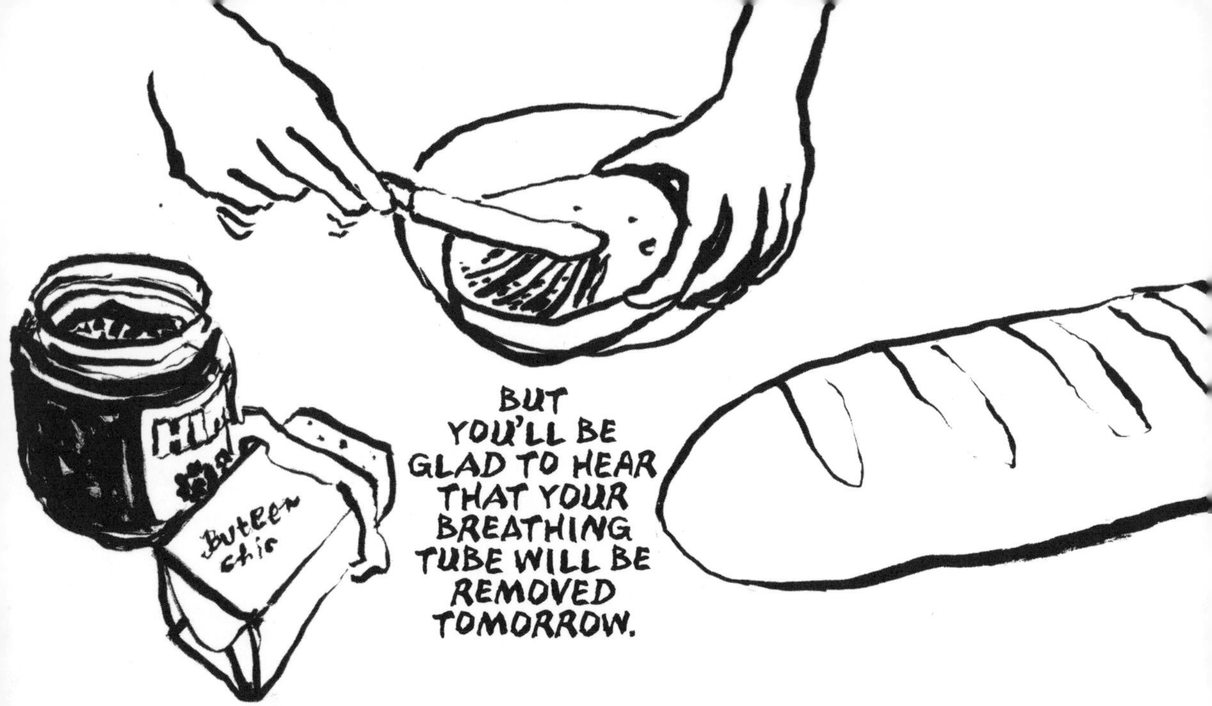
BUT YOU'LL BE GLAD TO HEAR THAT YOUR BREATHING TUBE WILL BE REMOVED TOMORROW.

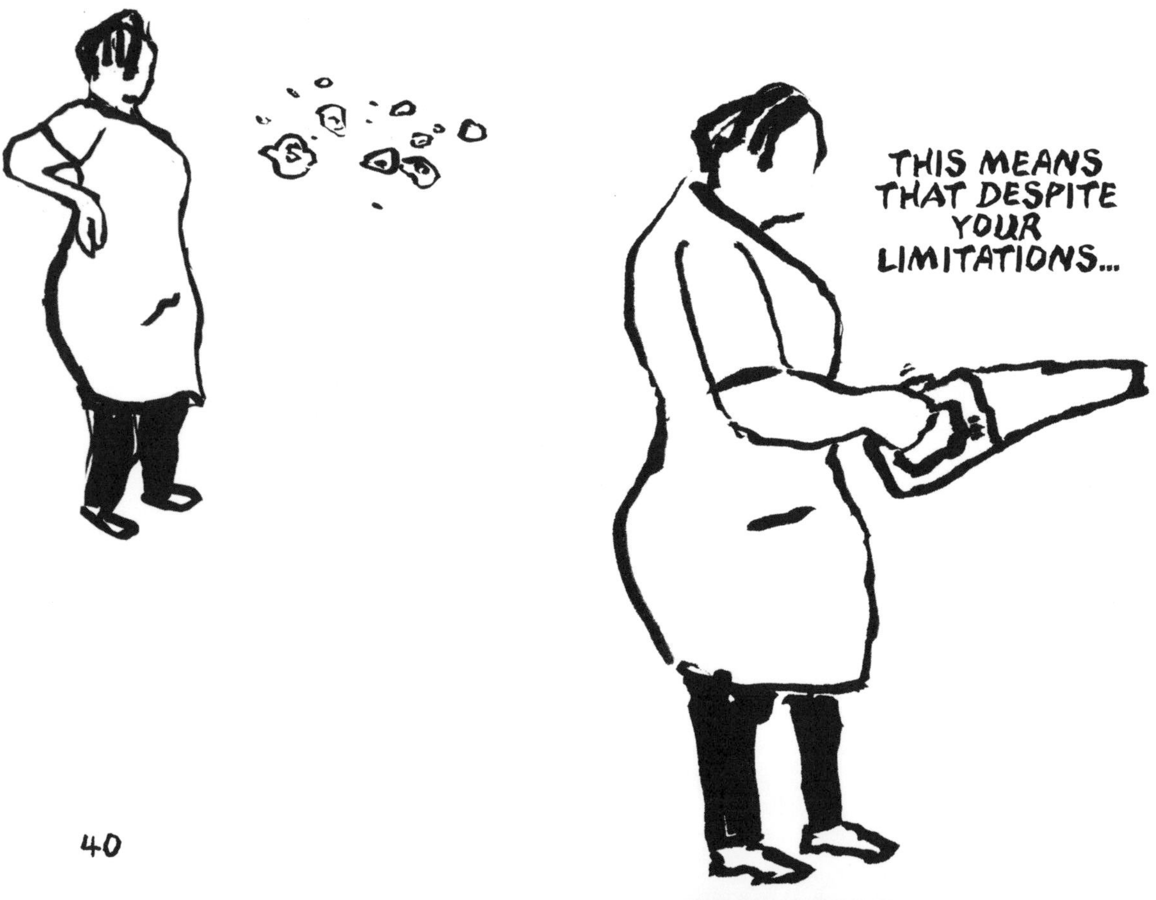
THIS MEANS THAT DESPITE YOUR LIMITATIONS...

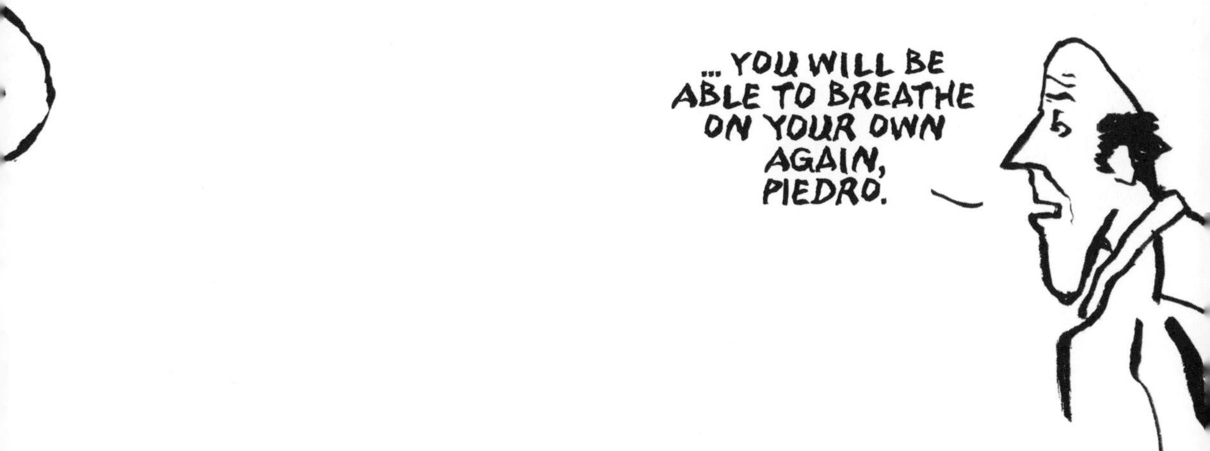
... YOU WILL BE ABLE TO BREATHE ON YOUR OWN AGAIN, PIEDRO.

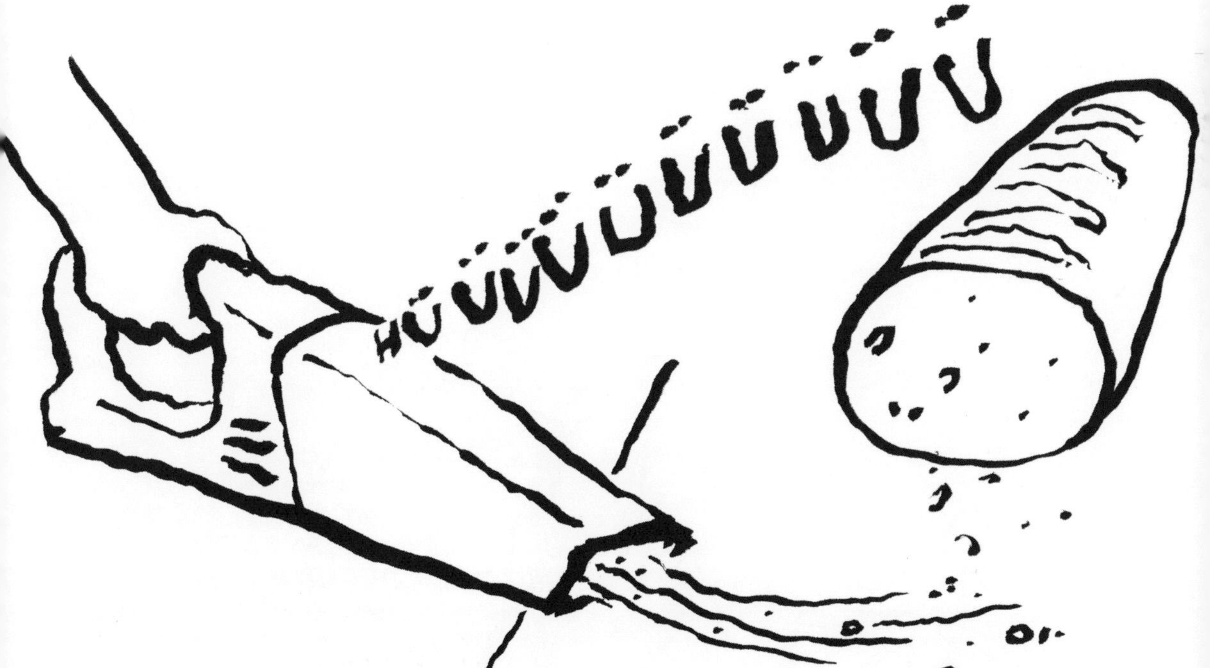

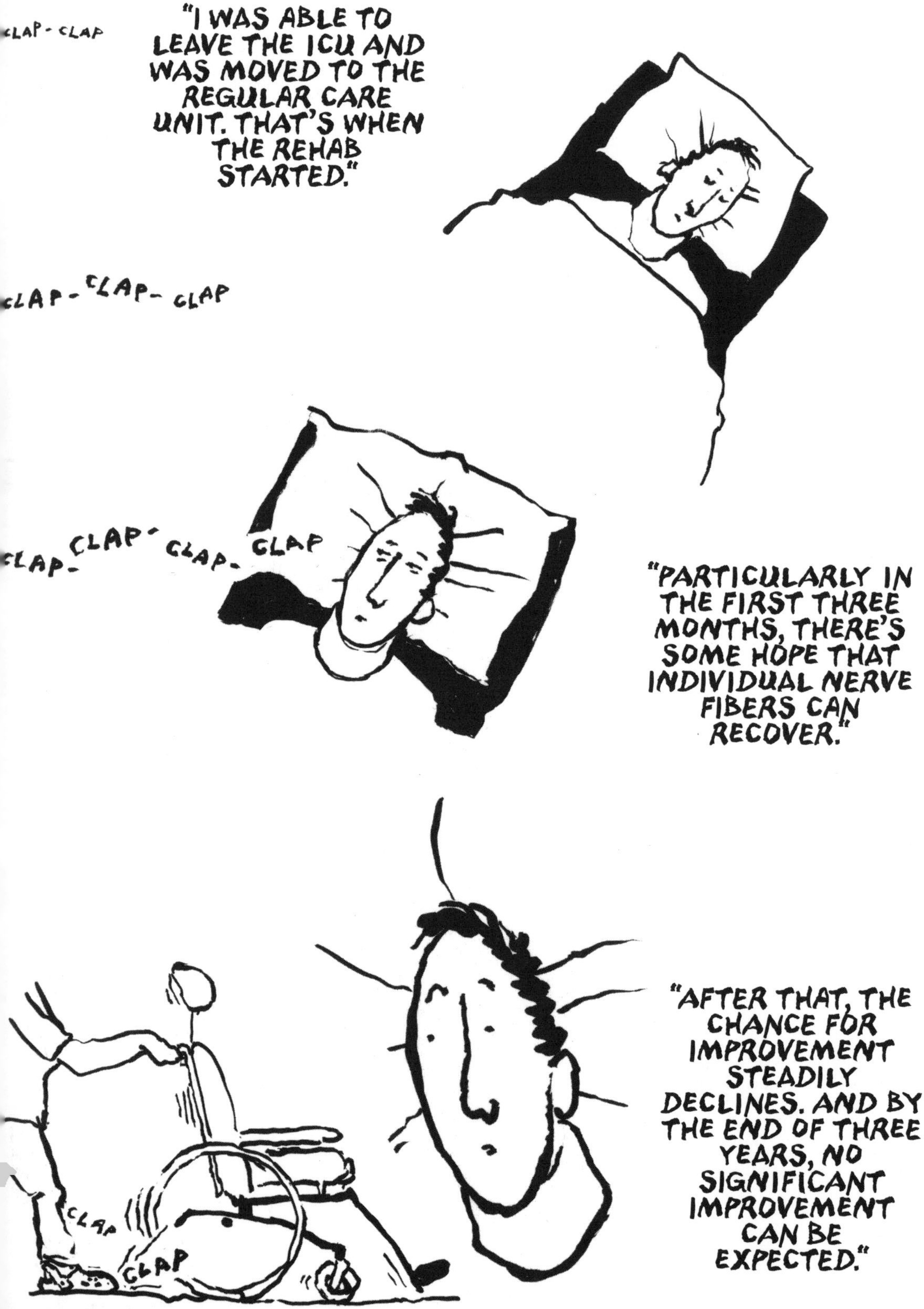
"I WAS ABLE TO LEAVE THE ICU AND WAS MOVED TO THE REGULAR CARE UNIT. THAT'S WHEN THE REHAB STARTED."
CLAP-CLAP
CLAP-CLAP-CLAP
CLAP-CLAP-CLAP-CLAP
"PARTICULARLY IN THE FIRST THREE MONTHS, THERE'S SOME HOPE THAT INDIVIDUAL NERVE FIBERS CAN RECOVER."
"AFTER THAT, THE CHANCE FOR IMPROVEMENT STEADILY DECLINES. AND BY THE END OF THREE YEARS, NO SIGNIFICANT IMPROVEMENT CAN BE EXPECTED."
CLAP
CLAP

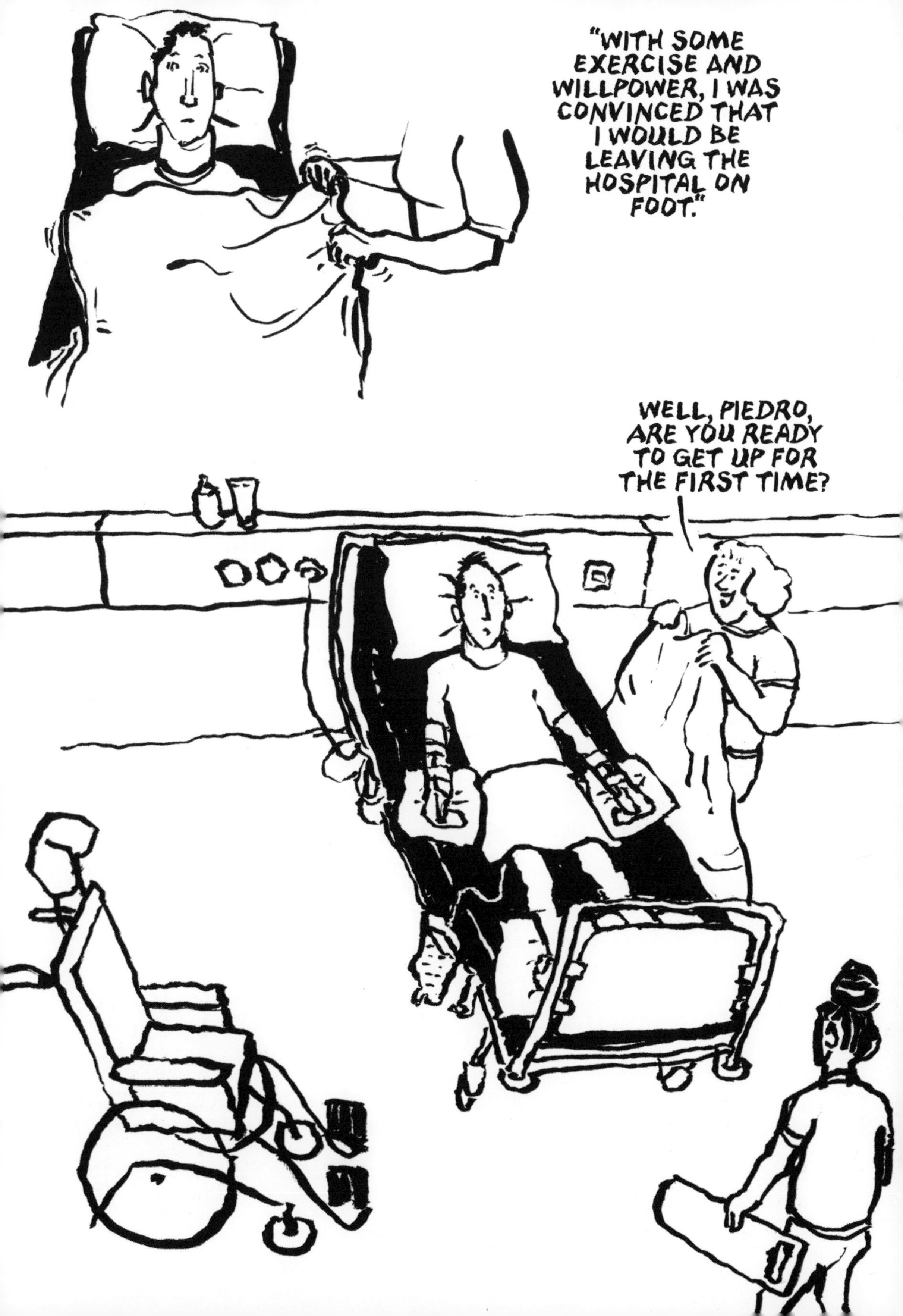
"WITH SOME EXERCISE AND WILLPOWER, I WAS CONVINCED THAT I WOULD BE LEAVING THE HOSPITAL ON FOOT."
WELL, PIEDRO, ARE YOU READY TO GET UP FOR THE FIRST TIME?

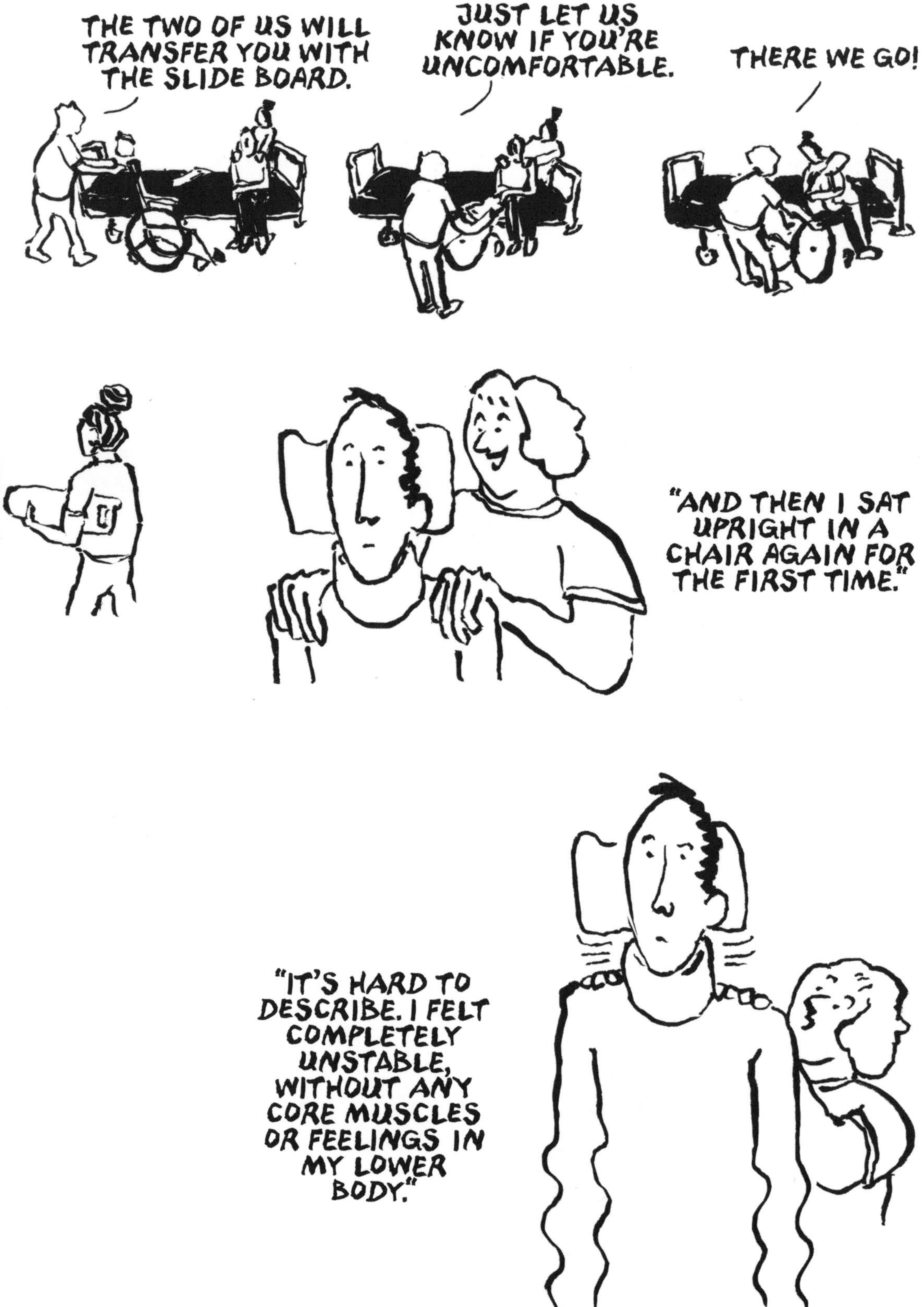
THE TWO OF US WILL TRANSFER YOU WITH THE SLIDE BOARD.
JUST LET US KNOW IF YOU'RE UNCOMFORTABLE.
THERE WE GO!
"AND THEN I SAT UPRIGHT IN A CHAIR AGAIN FOR THE FIRST TIME."
"IT'S HARD TO DESCRIBE. I FELT COMPLETELY UNSTABLE, WITHOUT ANY CORE MUSCLES OR FEELINGS IN MY LOWER BODY."

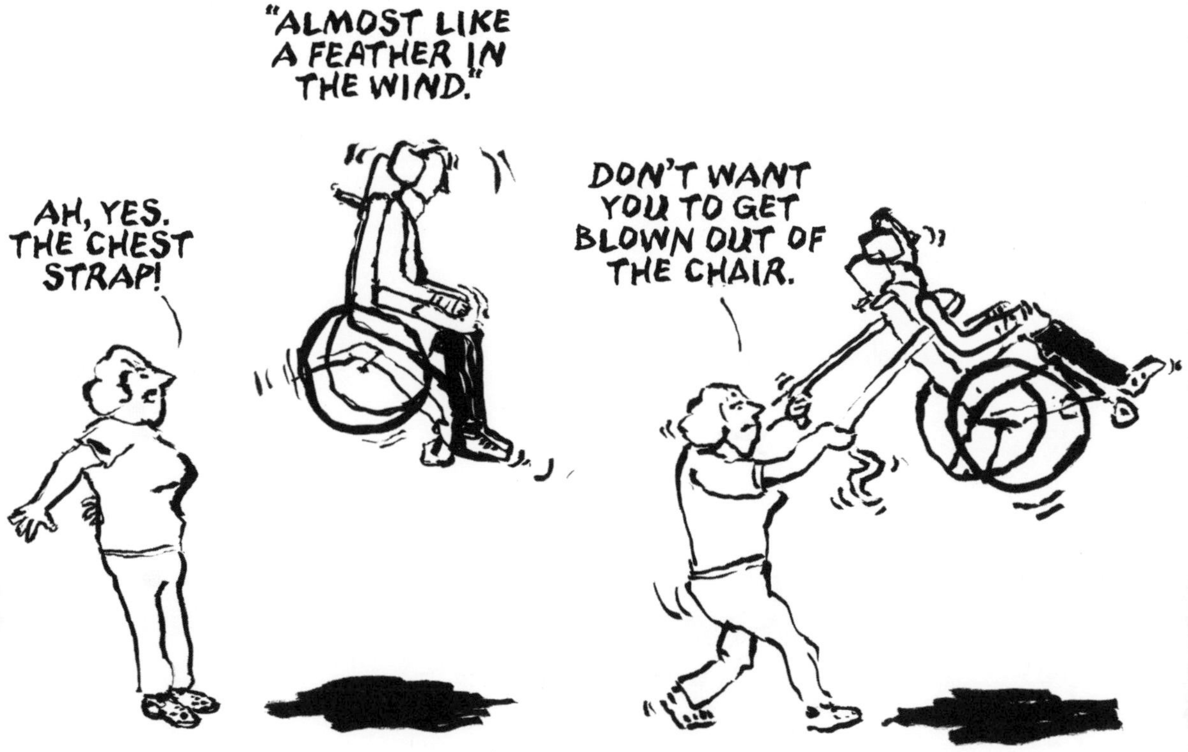
"ALMOST LIKE A FEATHER IN THE WIND."
AH, YES. THE CHEST STRAP!
DON'T WANT YOU TO GET BLOWN OUT OF THE CHAIR.

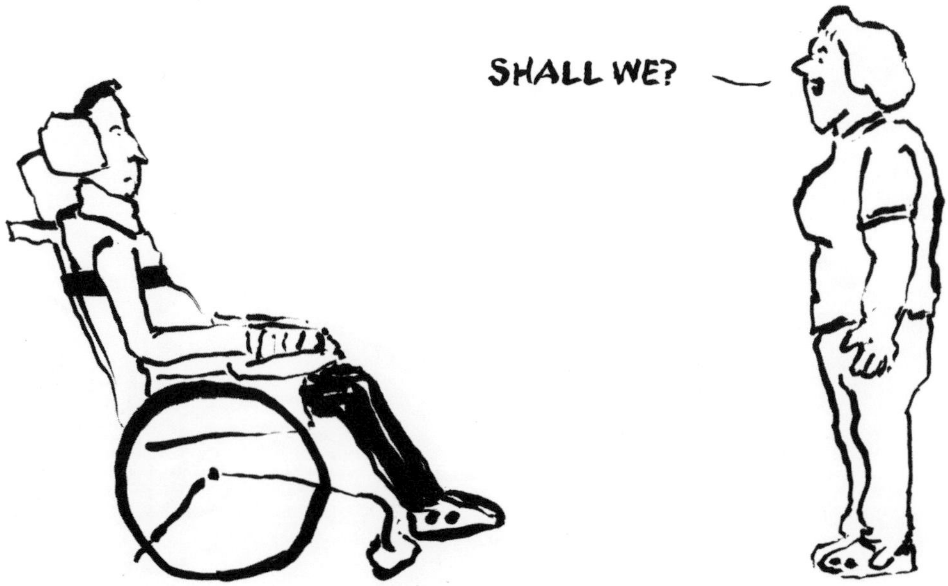
SHALL WE?

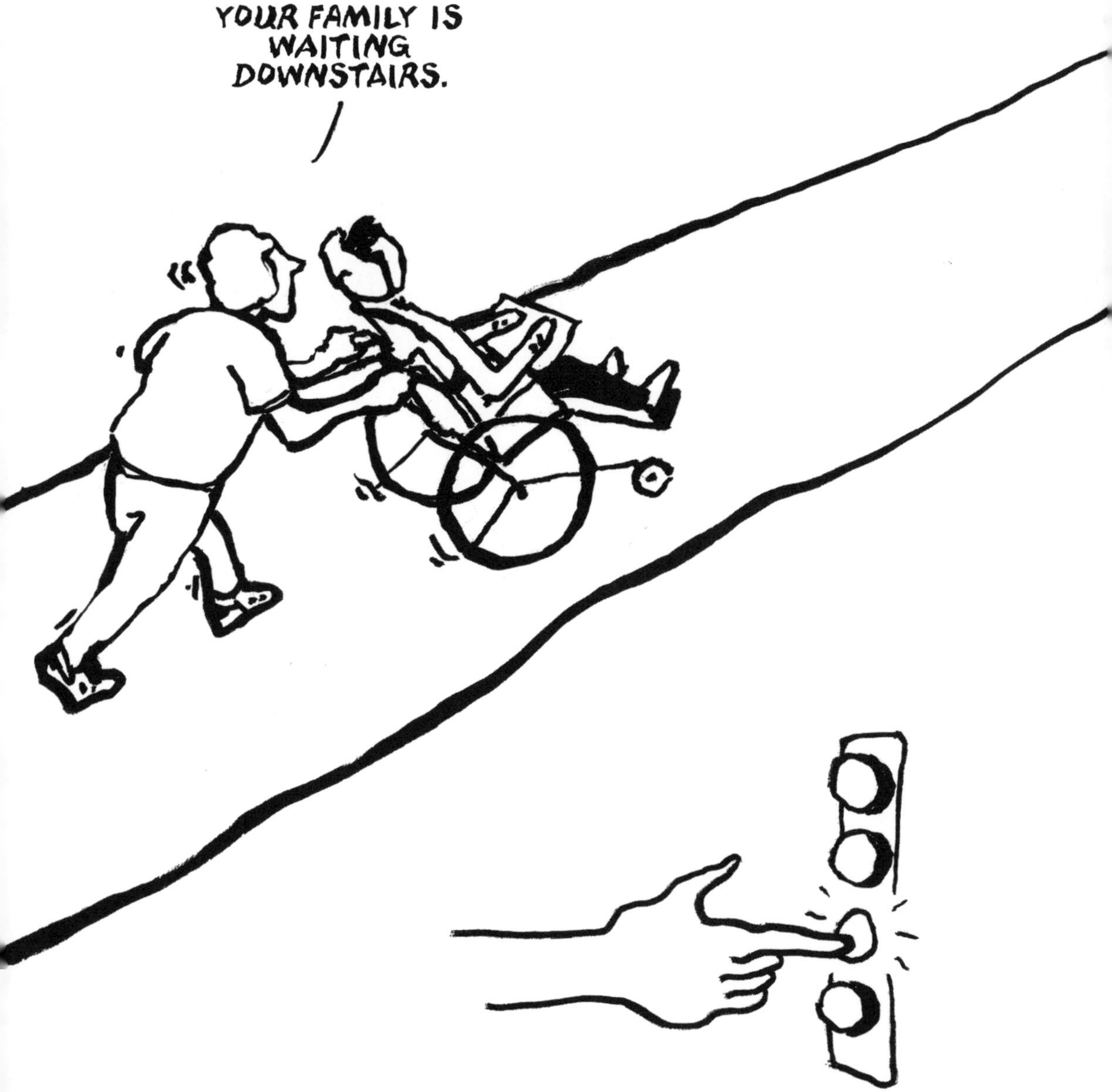
YOUR FAMILY IS WAITING DOWNSTAIRS.

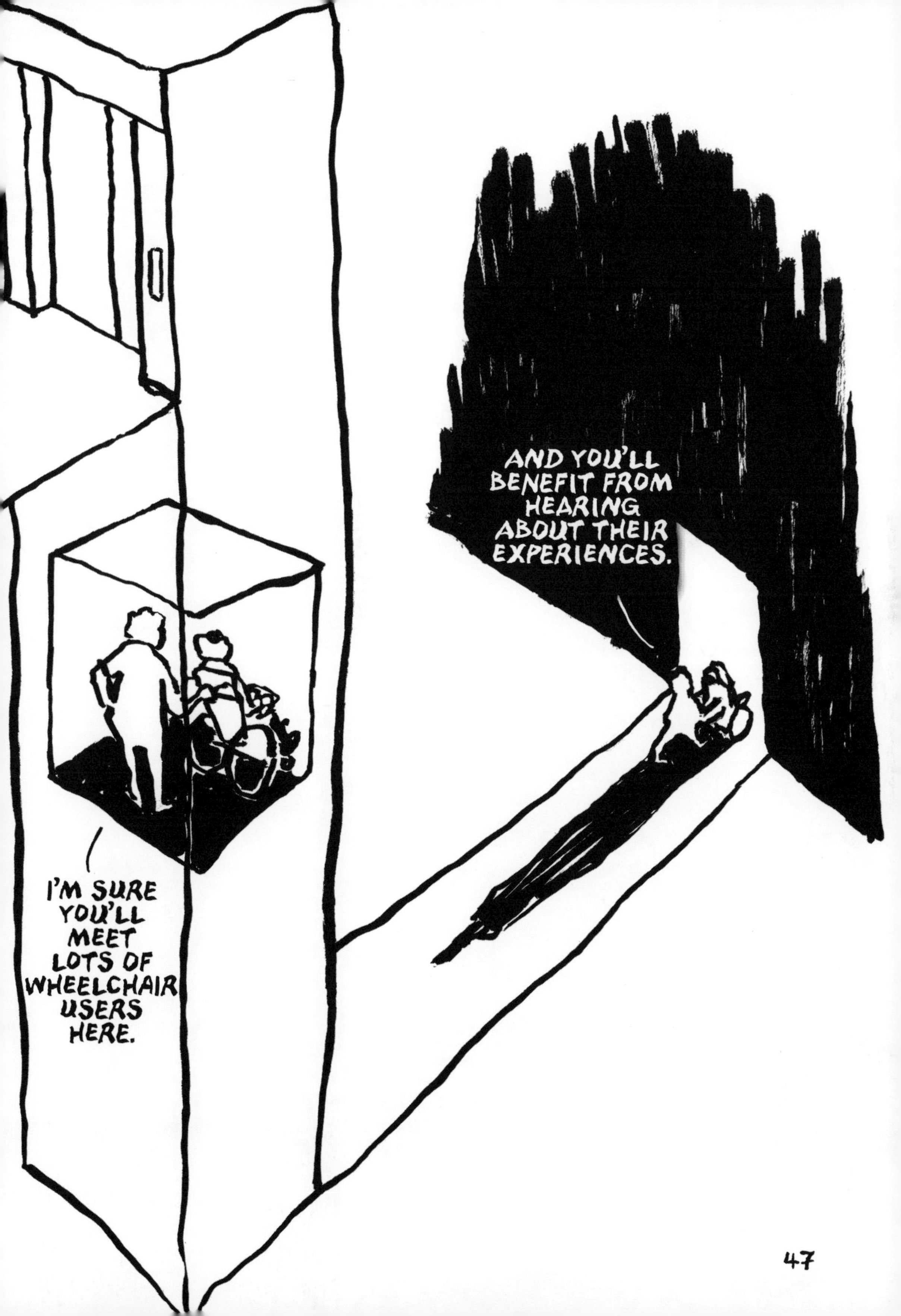
I'M SURE YOU'LL MEET LOTS OF WHEELCHAIR USERS HERE.
AND YOU'LL BENEFIT FROM HEARING ABOUT THEIR EXPERIENCES.

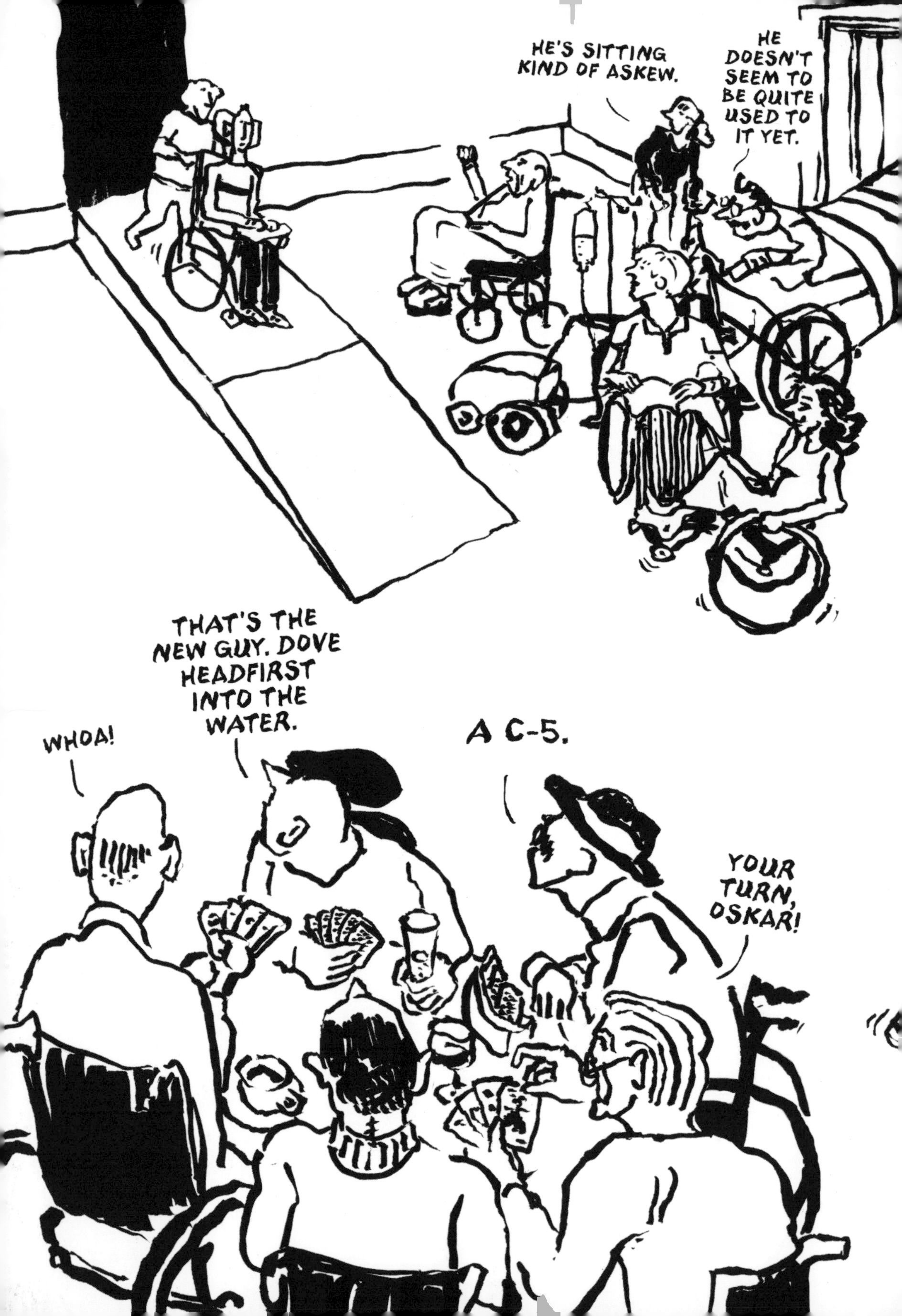
HE'S SITTING KIND OF ASKEW.
HE DOESN'T SEEM TO BE QUITE USED TO IT YET.
WHOA!
THAT'S THE NEW GUY. DOVE HEADFIRST INTO THE WATER.
A C-5.
YOUR TURN, OSKAR!

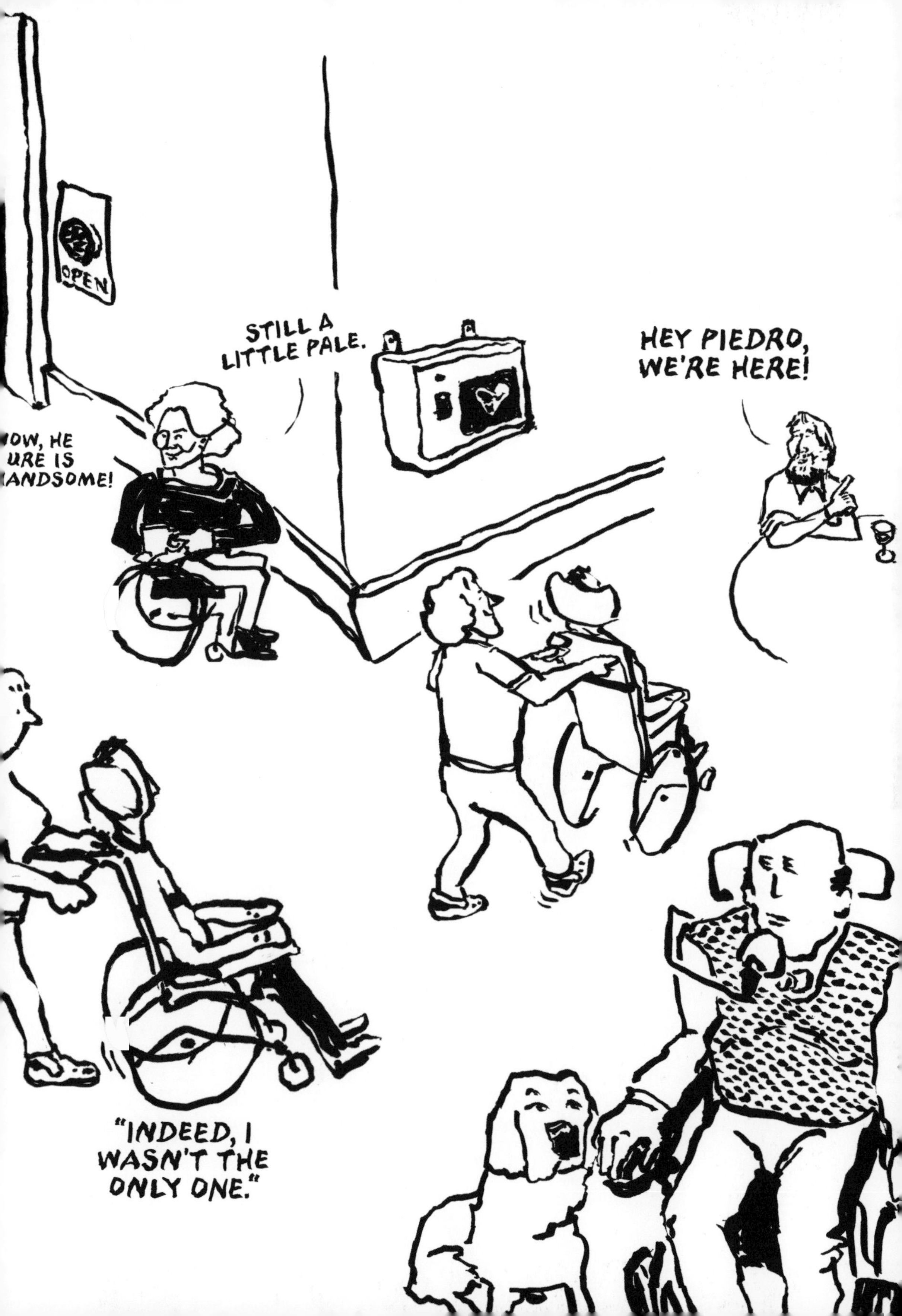
OPEN
OW, HE
URE IS
ANDSOME!
STILL A
LITTLE PALE.
HEY PIEDRO,
WE'RE HERE!
"INDEED, I
WASN'T THE
ONLY ONE."

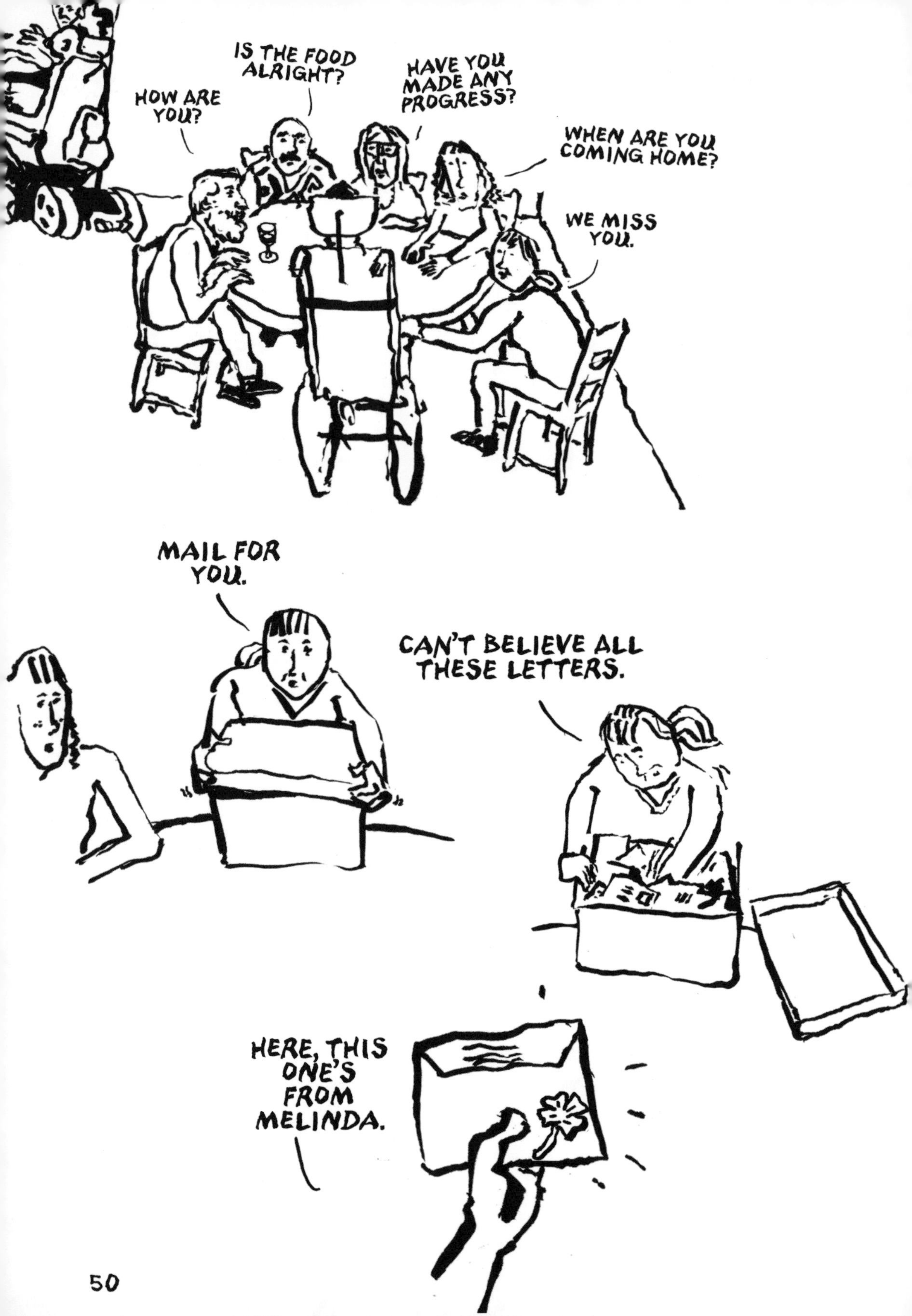
HOW ARE YOU?
IS THE FOOD ALRIGHT?
HAVE YOU MADE ANY PROGRESS?
WHEN ARE YOU COMING HOME?
WE MISS YOU.
MAIL FOR YOU.
CAN'T BELIEVE ALL THESE LETTERS.
HERE, THIS ONE'S FROM MELINDA.

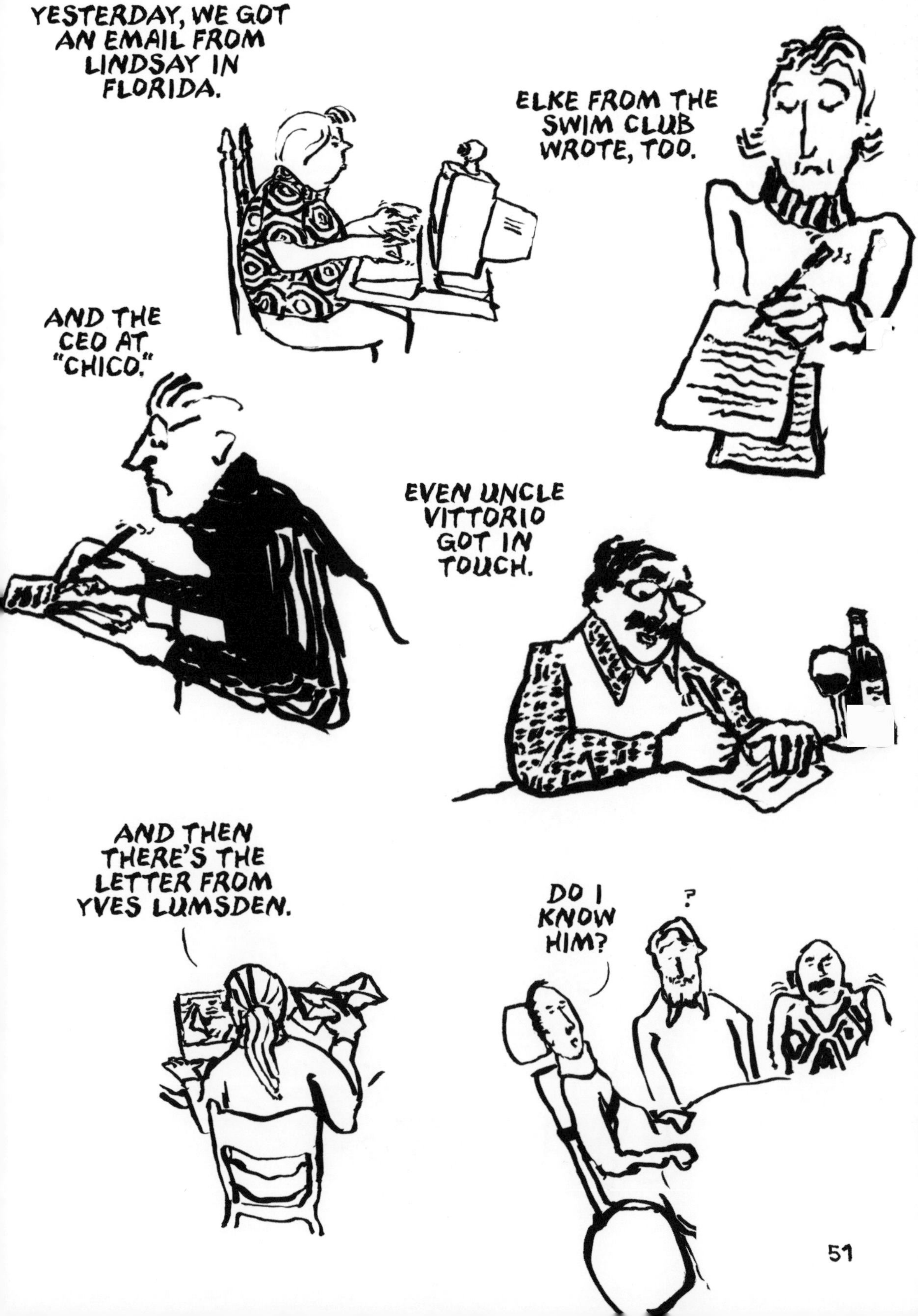
YESTERDAY, WE GOT AN EMAIL FROM LINDSAY IN FLORIDA.
ELKE FROM THE SWIM CLUB WROTE, TOO.
AND THE CEO AT "CHICO."
EVEN UNCLE VITTORIO GOT IN TOUCH.
AND THEN THERE'S THE LETTER FROM YVES LUMSDEN.
?
DO I KNOW HIM?

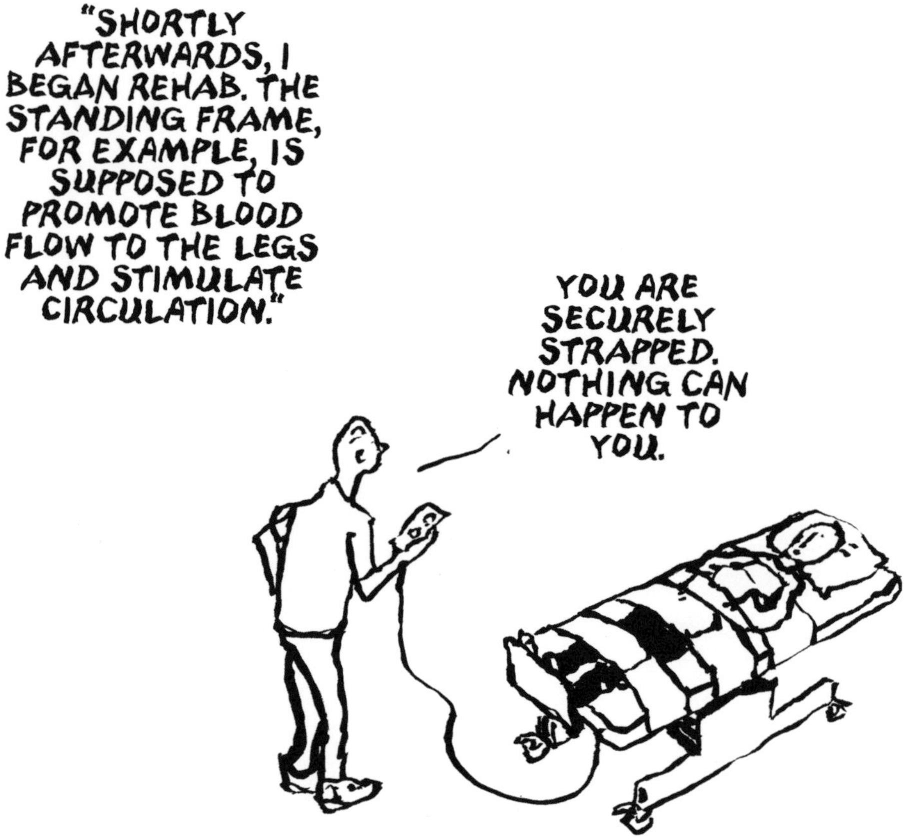
"SHORTLY AFTERWARDS, I BEGAN REHAB. THE STANDING FRAME, FOR EXAMPLE, IS SUPPOSED TO PROMOTE BLOOD FLOW TO THE LEGS AND STIMULATE CIRCULATION."
YOU ARE SECURELY STRAPPED. NOTHING CAN HAPPEN TO YOU.

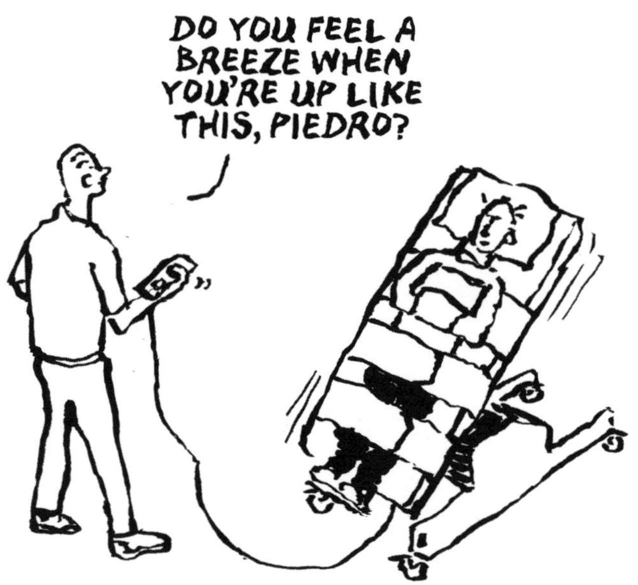
DO YOU FEEL A BREEZE WHEN YOU'RE UP LIKE THIS, PIEDRO?

I'LL BE
RIGHT
BACK.

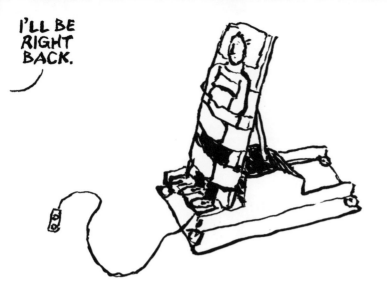

"I FELT A CALM
RISE WITHIN ME.
IT REALLY WAS
LIBERATING."

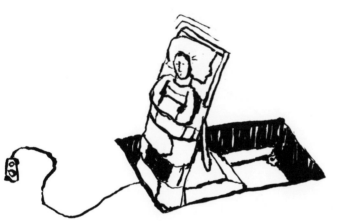

"AND THEN I
DISAPPEARED."

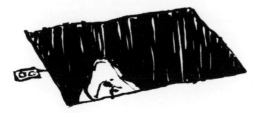

PIEEEDRO, ARE YOU DOWN THERE?

COME BACK!

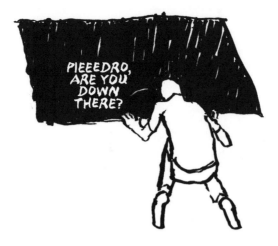

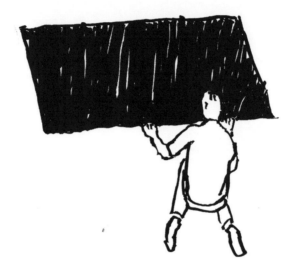

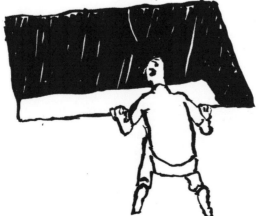

WHAT ARE YOU DOING?

FEELING BETTER?
DRINK THIS, YOU NEED SUGAR!
chico cola

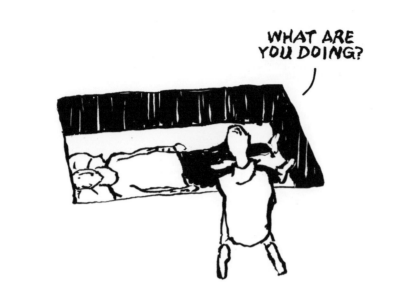

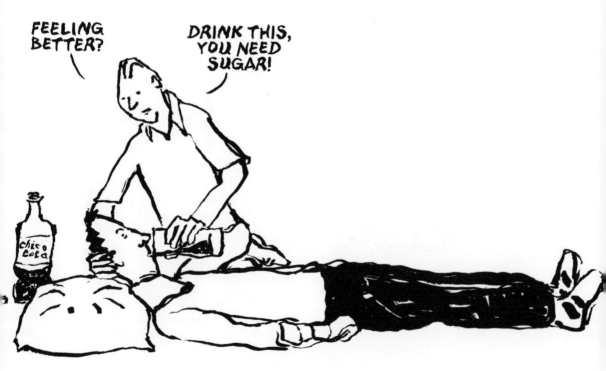

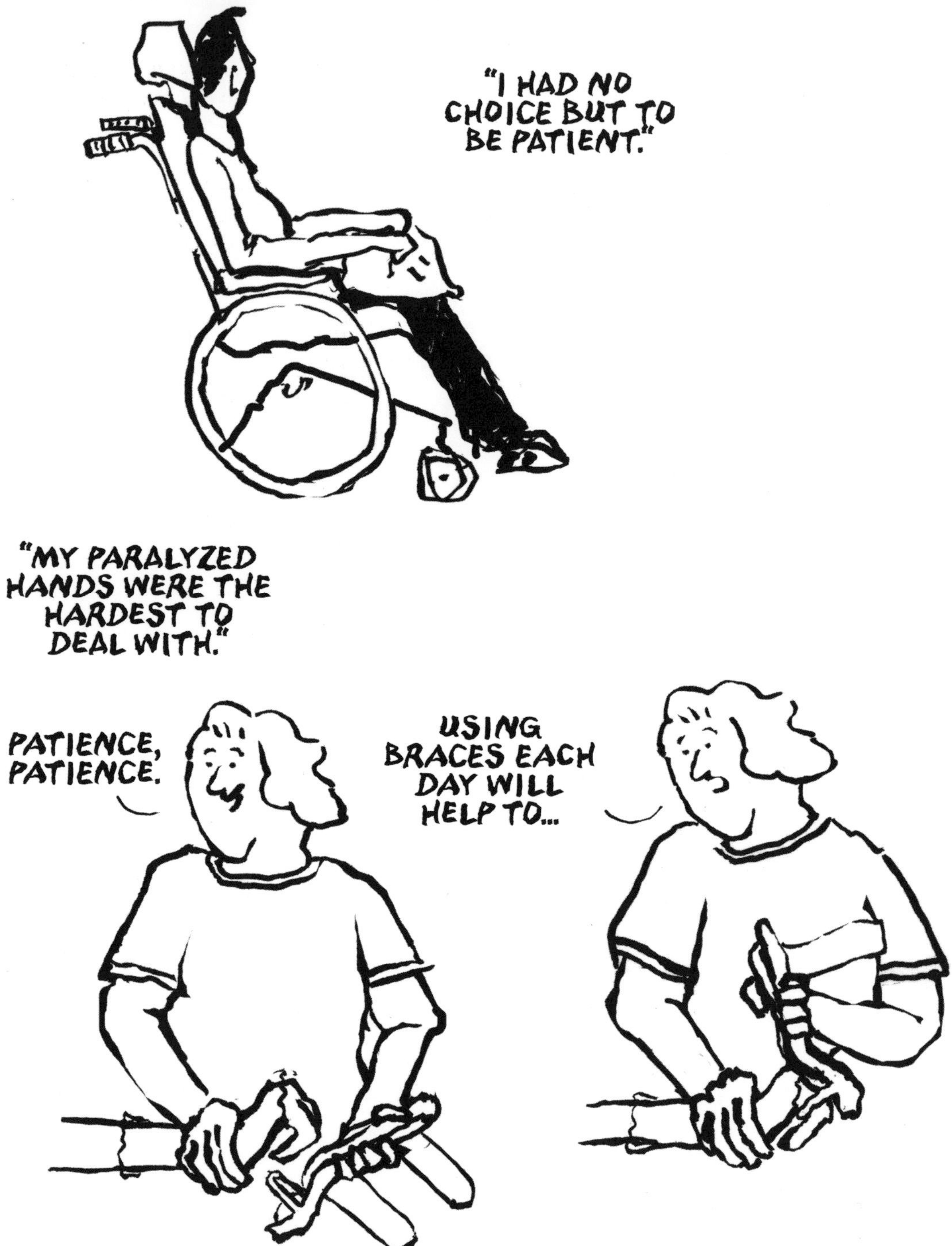
"I HAD NO CHOICE BUT TO BE PATIENT."
"MY PARALYZED HANDS WERE THE HARDEST TO DEAL WITH."
PATIENCE, PATIENCE.
USING BRACES EACH DAY WILL HELP TO...
KEEP YOUR FINGERS IN THIS BENT POSITION.

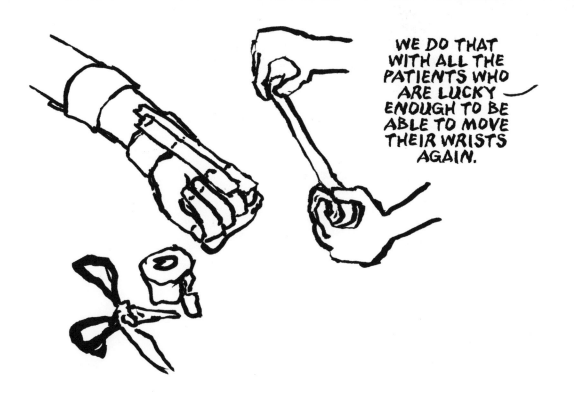

WE DO THAT WITH ALL THE PATIENTS WHO ARE LUCKY ENOUGH TO BE ABLE TO MOVE THEIR WRISTS AGAIN.

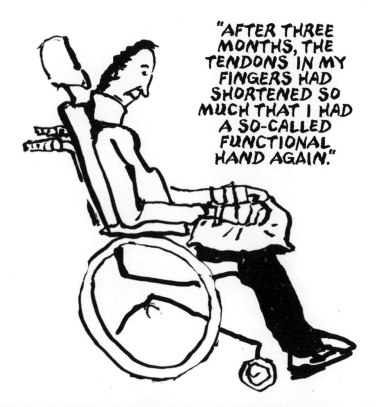

"AFTER THREE MONTHS, THE TENDONS IN MY FINGERS HAD SHORTENED SO MUCH THAT I HAD A SO-CALLED FUNCTIONAL HAND AGAIN."

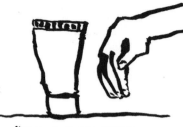

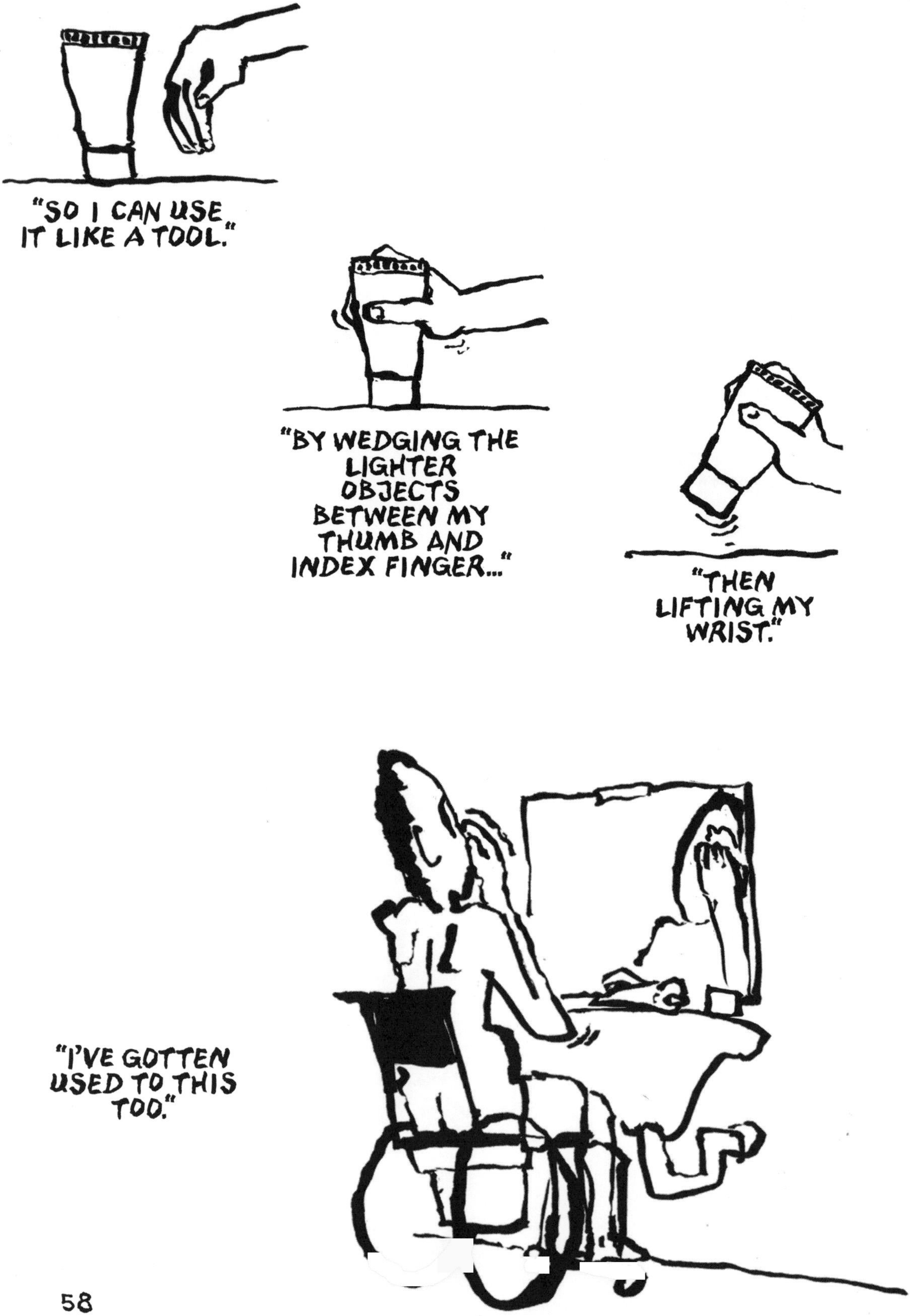

"SO I CAN USE IT LIKE A TOOL."

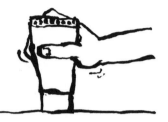

"BY WEDGING THE LIGHTER OBJECTS BETWEEN MY THUMB AND INDEX FINGER..."

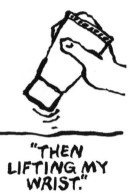

"THEN LIFTING MY WRIST."

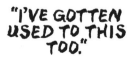

"I'VE GOTTEN USED TO THIS TOO."

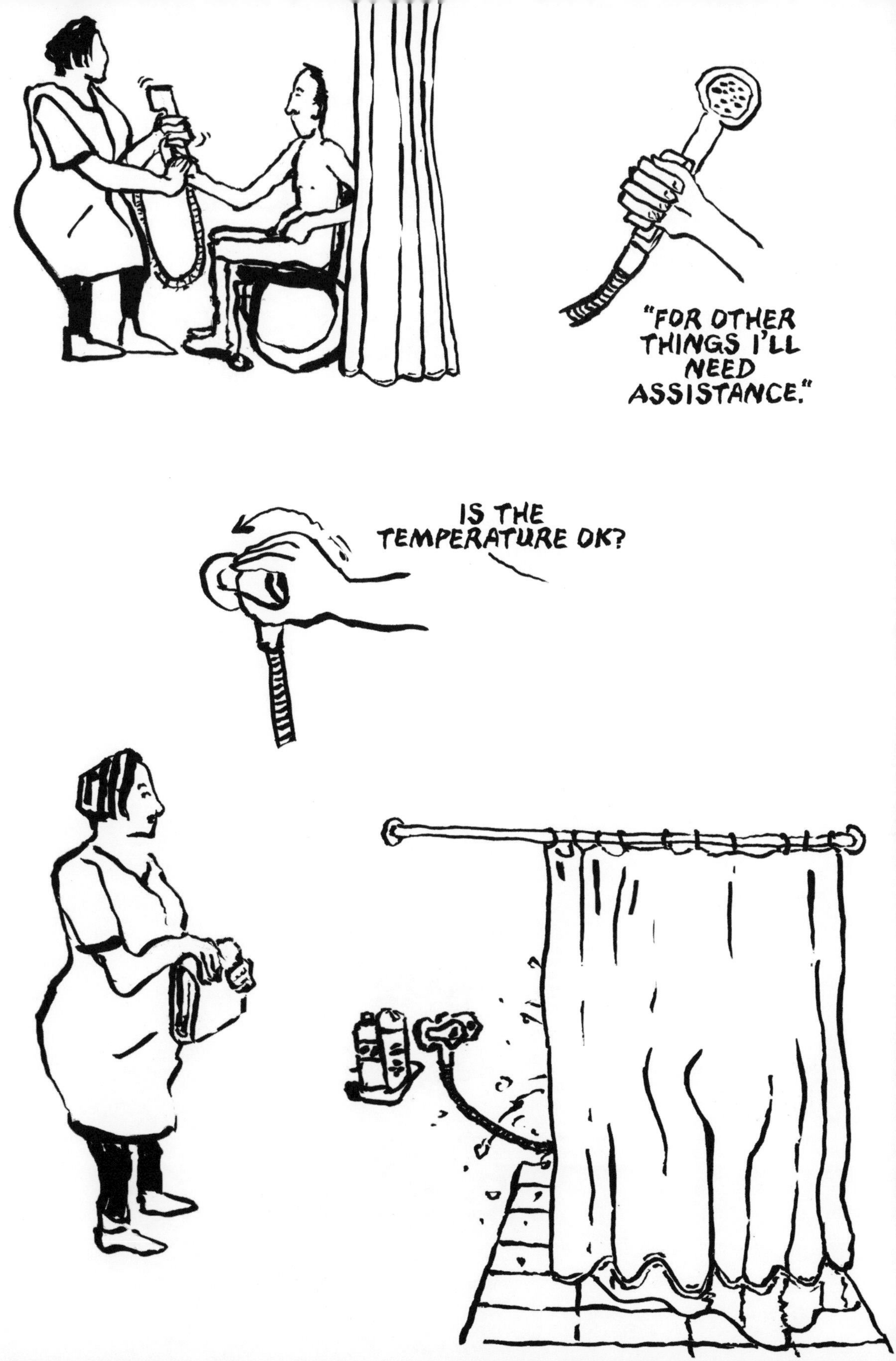
"FOR OTHER THINGS I'LL NEED ASSISTANCE."
IS THE TEMPERATURE OK?

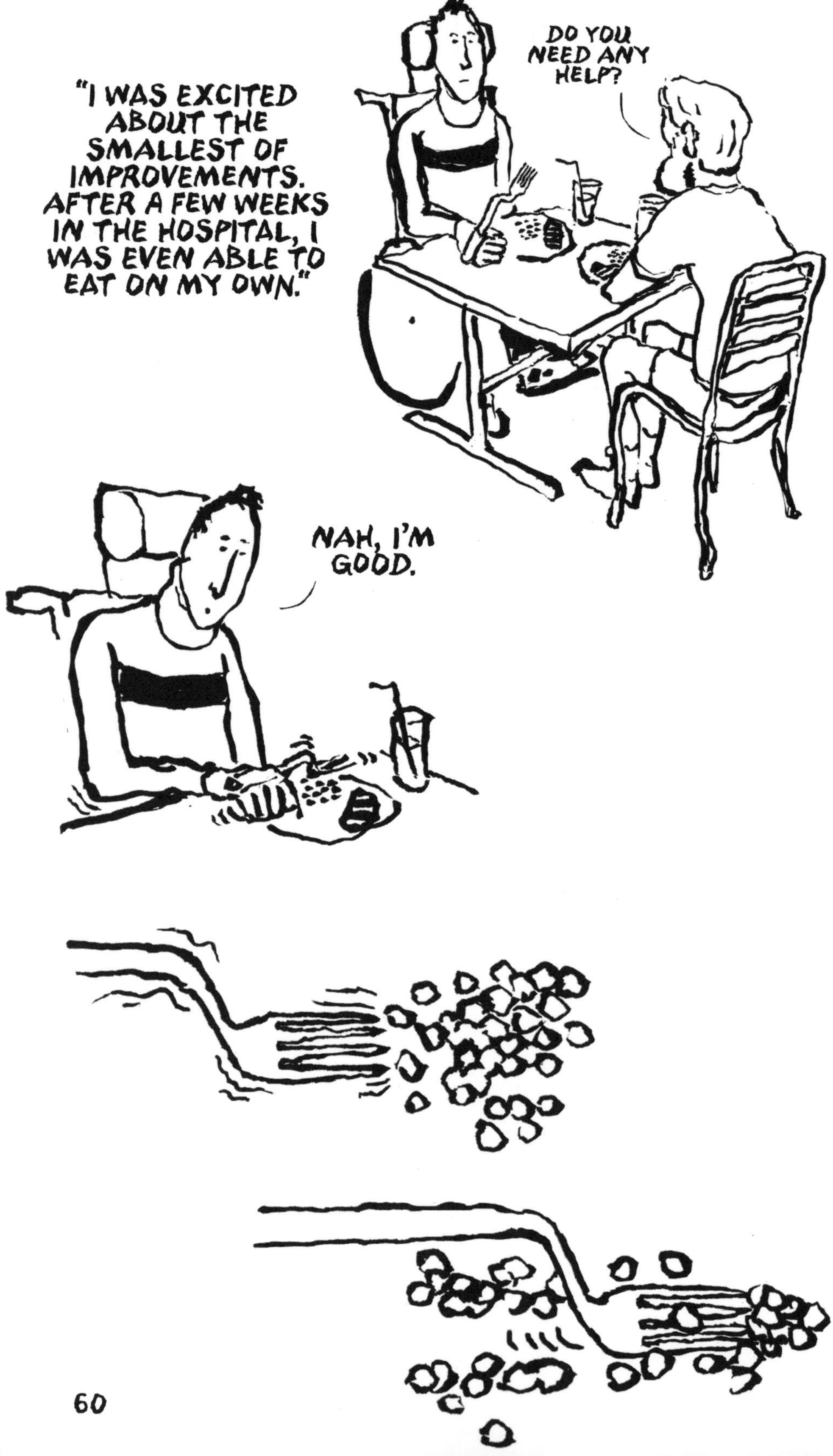

"I WAS EXCITED ABOUT THE SMALLEST OF IMPROVEMENTS. AFTER A FEW WEEKS IN THE HOSPITAL, I WAS EVEN ABLE TO EAT ON MY OWN."
DO YOU NEED ANY HELP?
NAH, I'M GOOD.

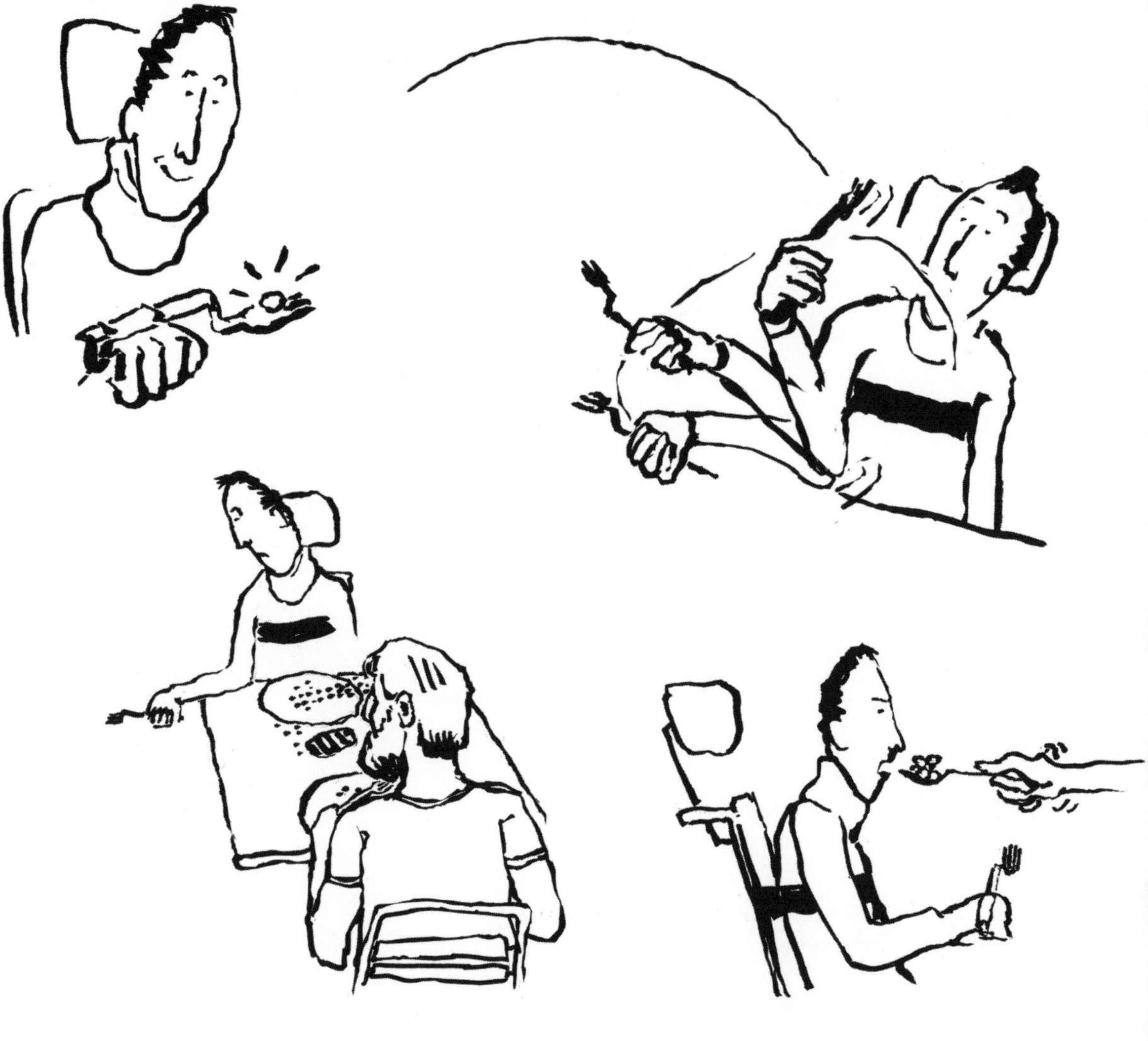
"THE NECK BRACE CAME OFF SOON. MY MUSCLES GOT STRONGER, BUT NOTHING CHANGED ABOUT THE EXTENT OF MY PARALYSIS."

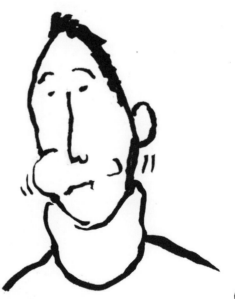

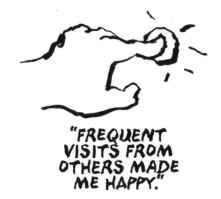

"FREQUENT VISITS FROM OTHERS MADE ME HAPPY."

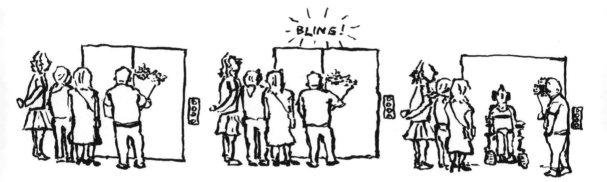

BLING!

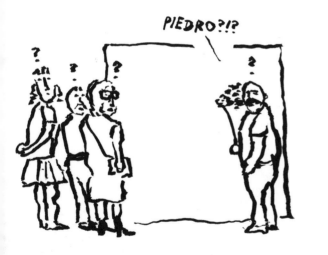

PIEDRO?!?

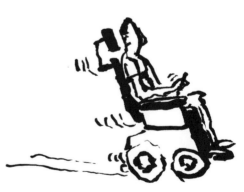

"BUT IN TIME I ALSO NEEDED SPACE."

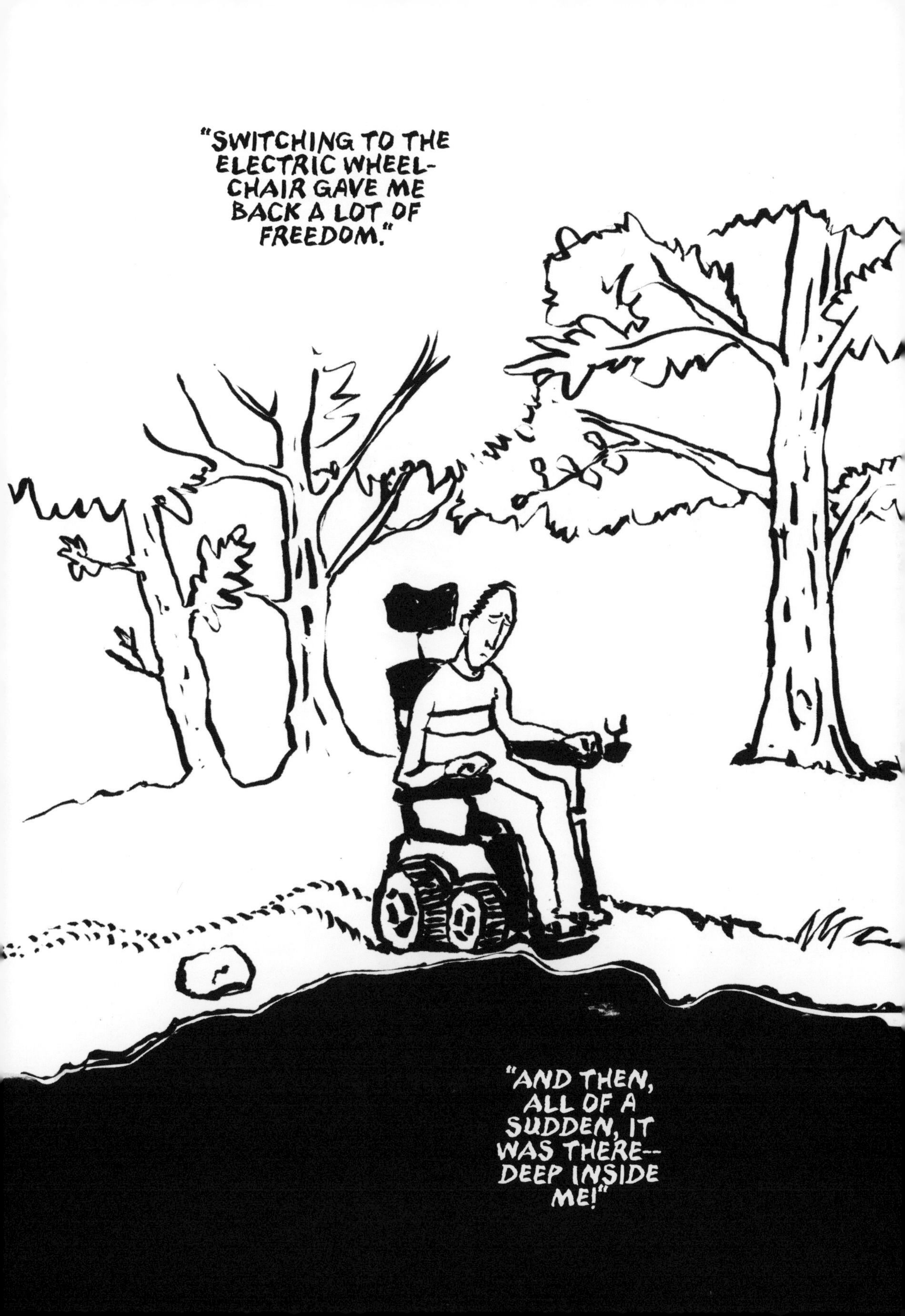
"SWITCHING TO THE ELECTRIC WHEEL-CHAIR GAVE ME BACK A LOT OF FREEDOM."
"AND THEN, ALL OF A SUDDEN, IT WAS THERE-- DEEP INSIDE ME!"

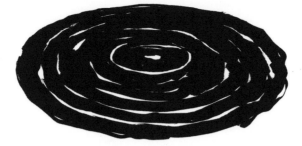

"STARING UP AT ME
FROM THE ABYSS."

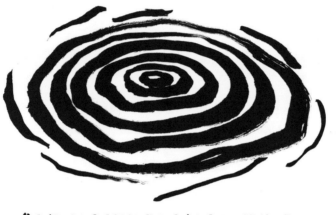

"THE CERTAINTY THAT I WOULD
BE PARALYZED FOREVER."

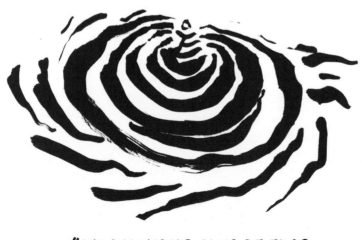

"AN OMINOUS MIX OF FEAR
AND POWERLESSNESS..."

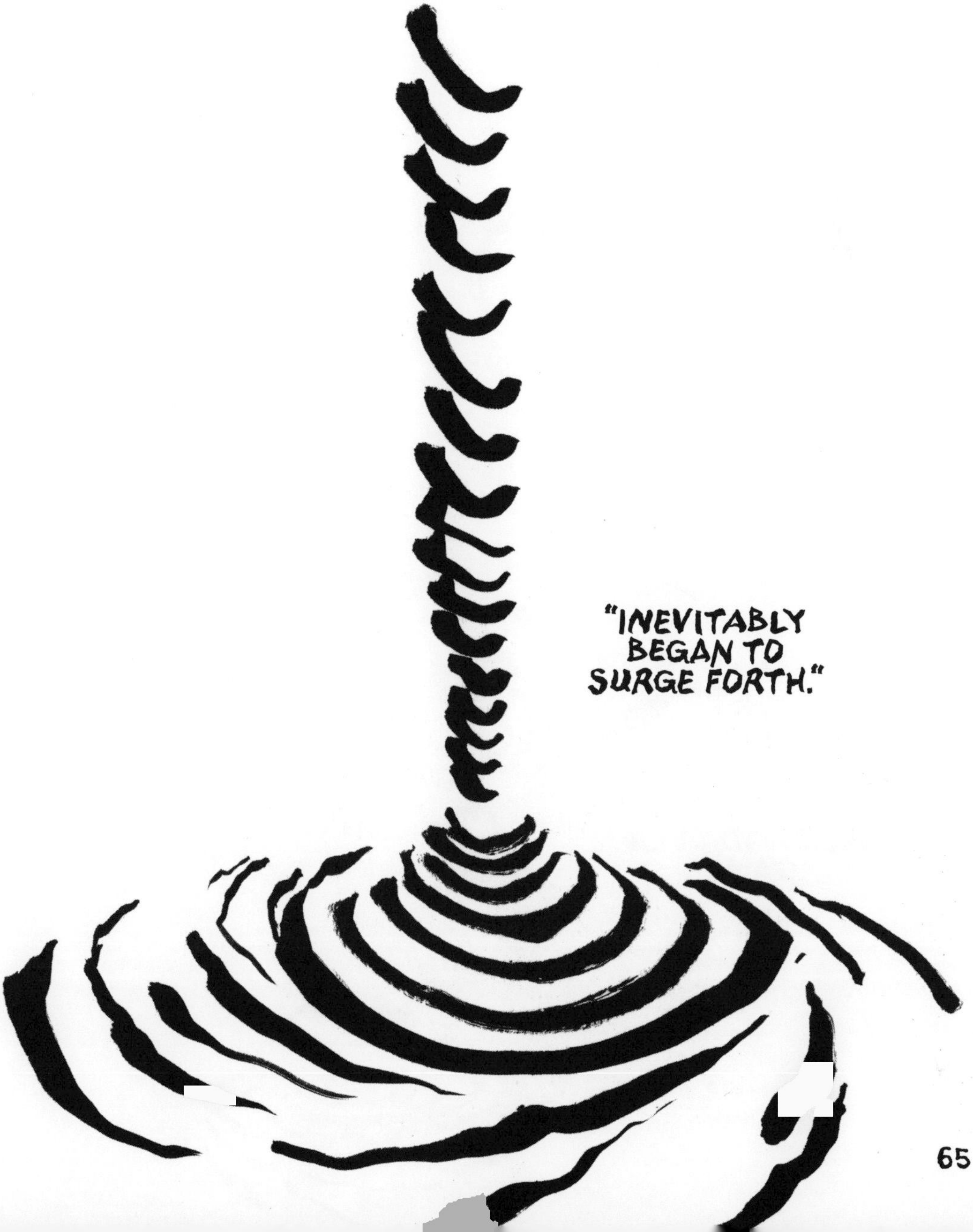
"INEVITABLY BEGAN TO SURGE FORTH."

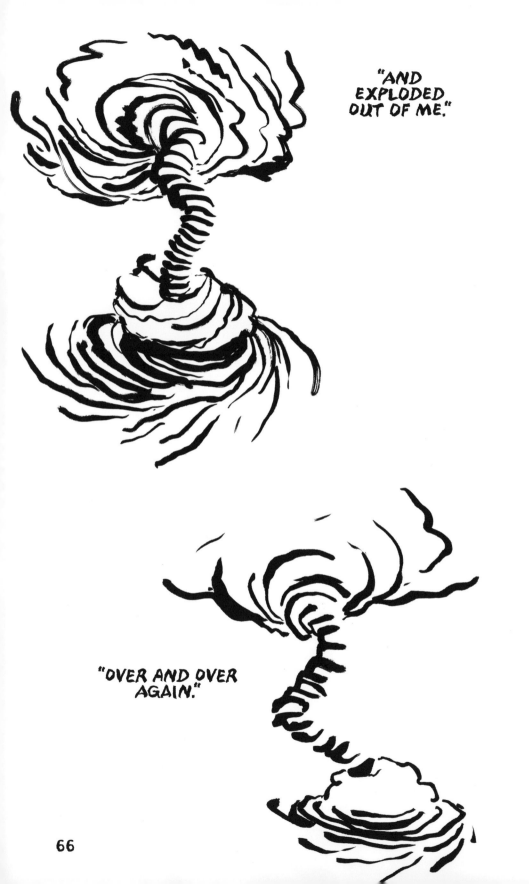

"AND EXPLODED OUT OF ME."

"OVER AND OVER AGAIN."

"UNTIL I HAD RESIGNED MYSELF TO IT."

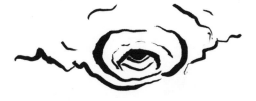

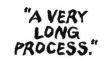

"A VERY LONG PROCESS."

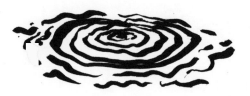

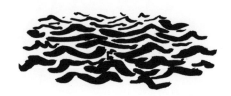

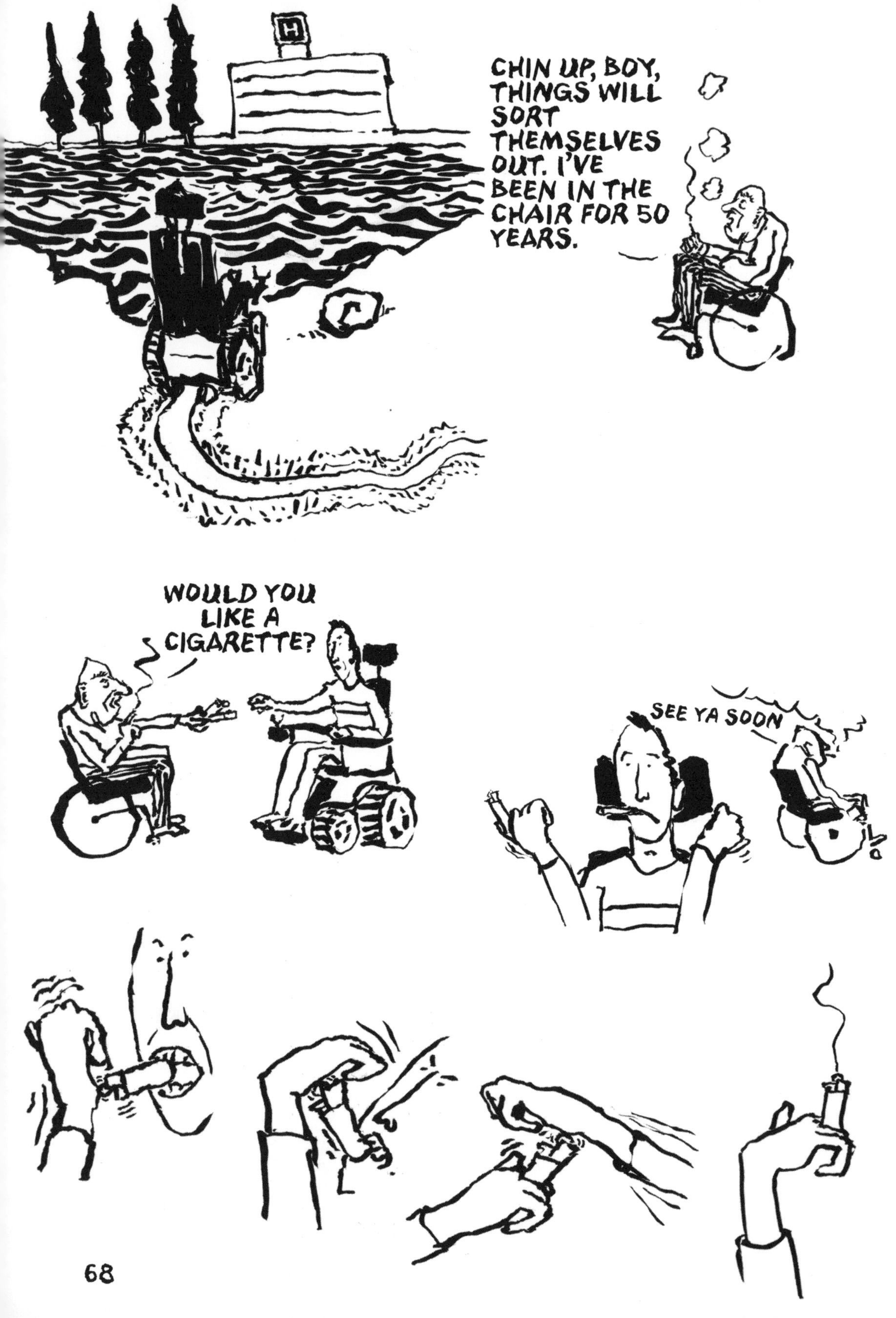
CHIN UP, BOY, THINGS WILL SORT THEMSELVES OUT. I'VE BEEN IN THE CHAIR FOR 50 YEARS.
WOULD YOU LIKE A CIGARETTE?
SEE YA SOON

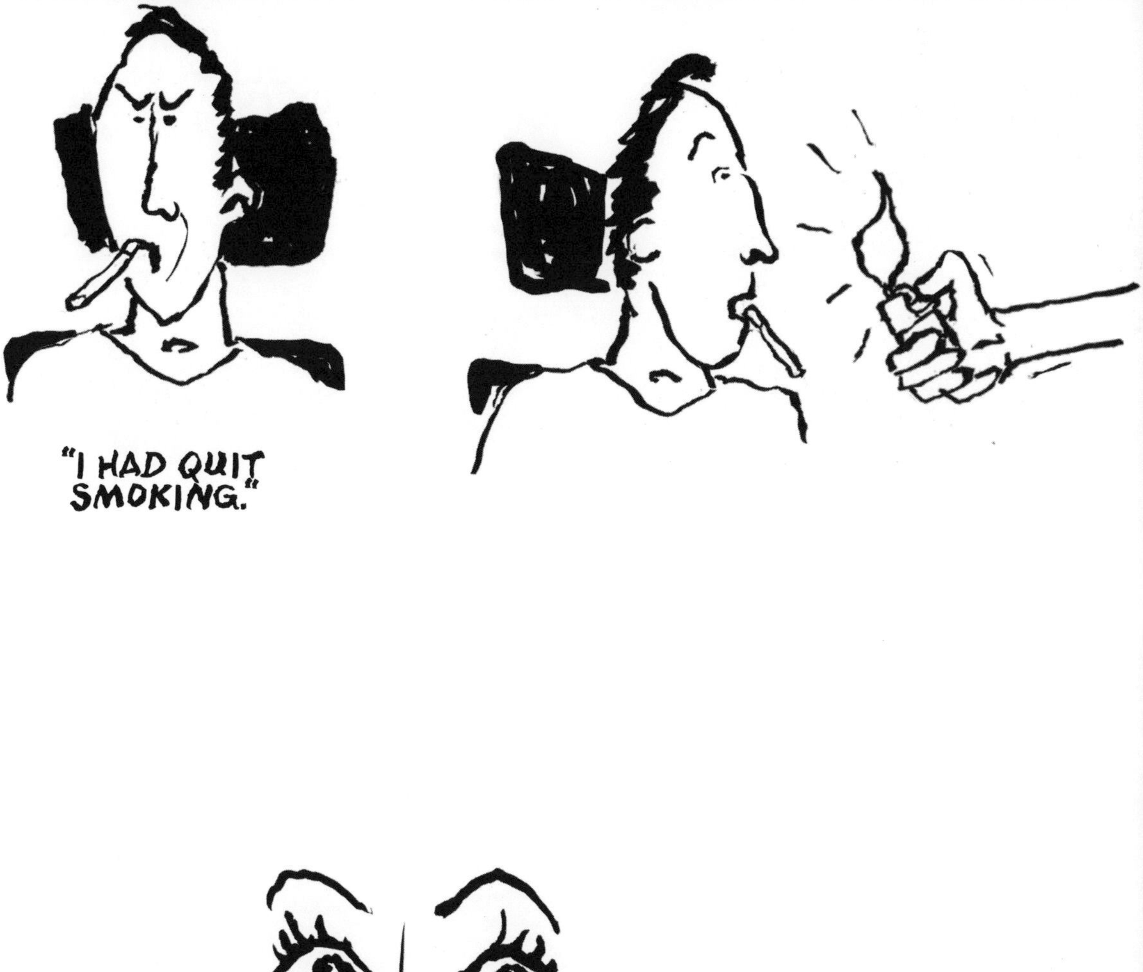
"I HAD QUIT SMOKING."
"BUT THEN I MET CHARLOTTE. MY PHYSICAL THERAPIST."

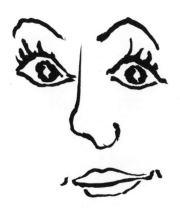

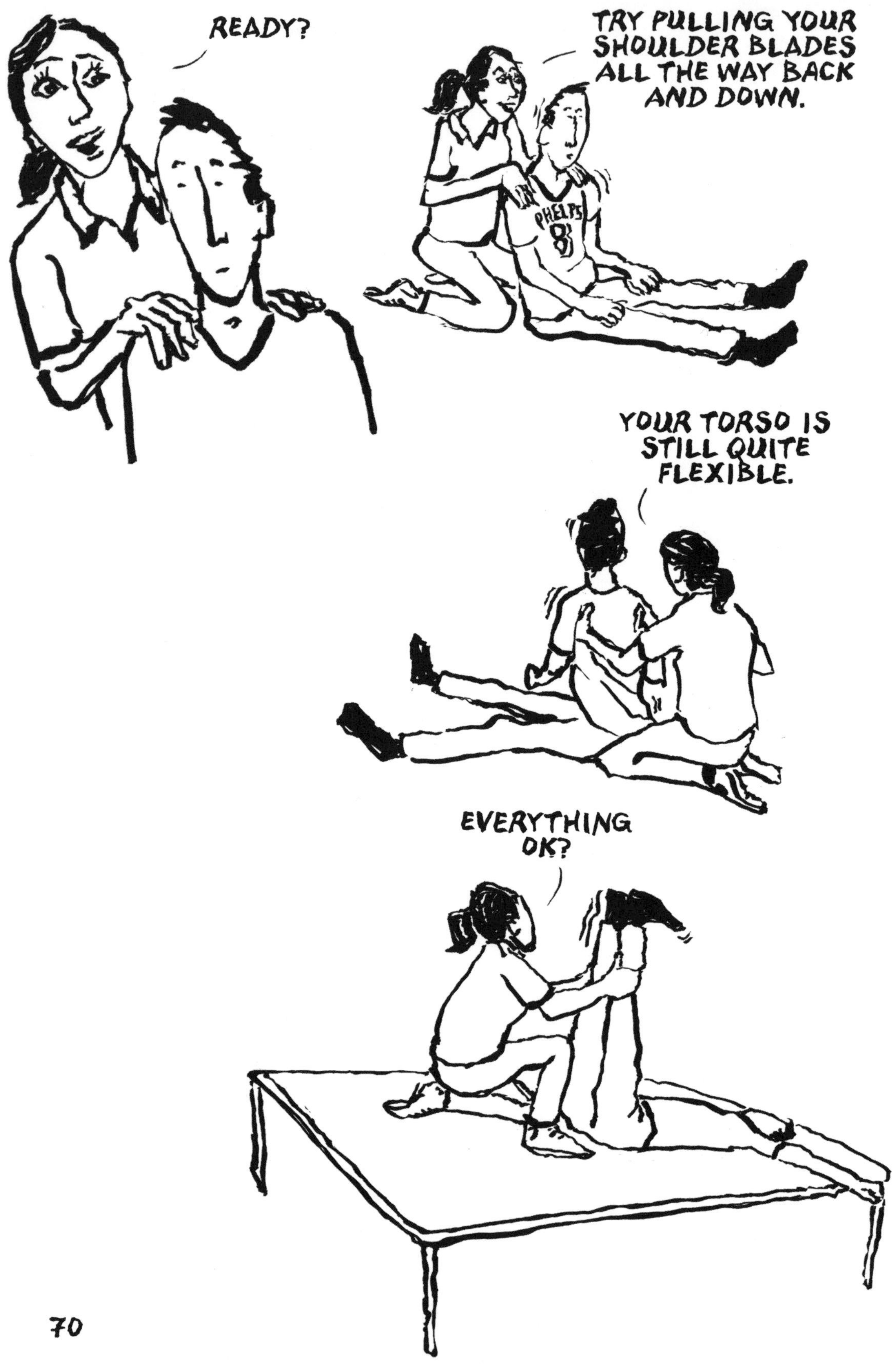
READY?
TRY PULLING YOUR SHOULDER BLADES ALL THE WAY BACK AND DOWN.
PHELPS 8
YOUR TORSO IS STILL QUITE FLEXIBLE.
EVERYTHING OK?

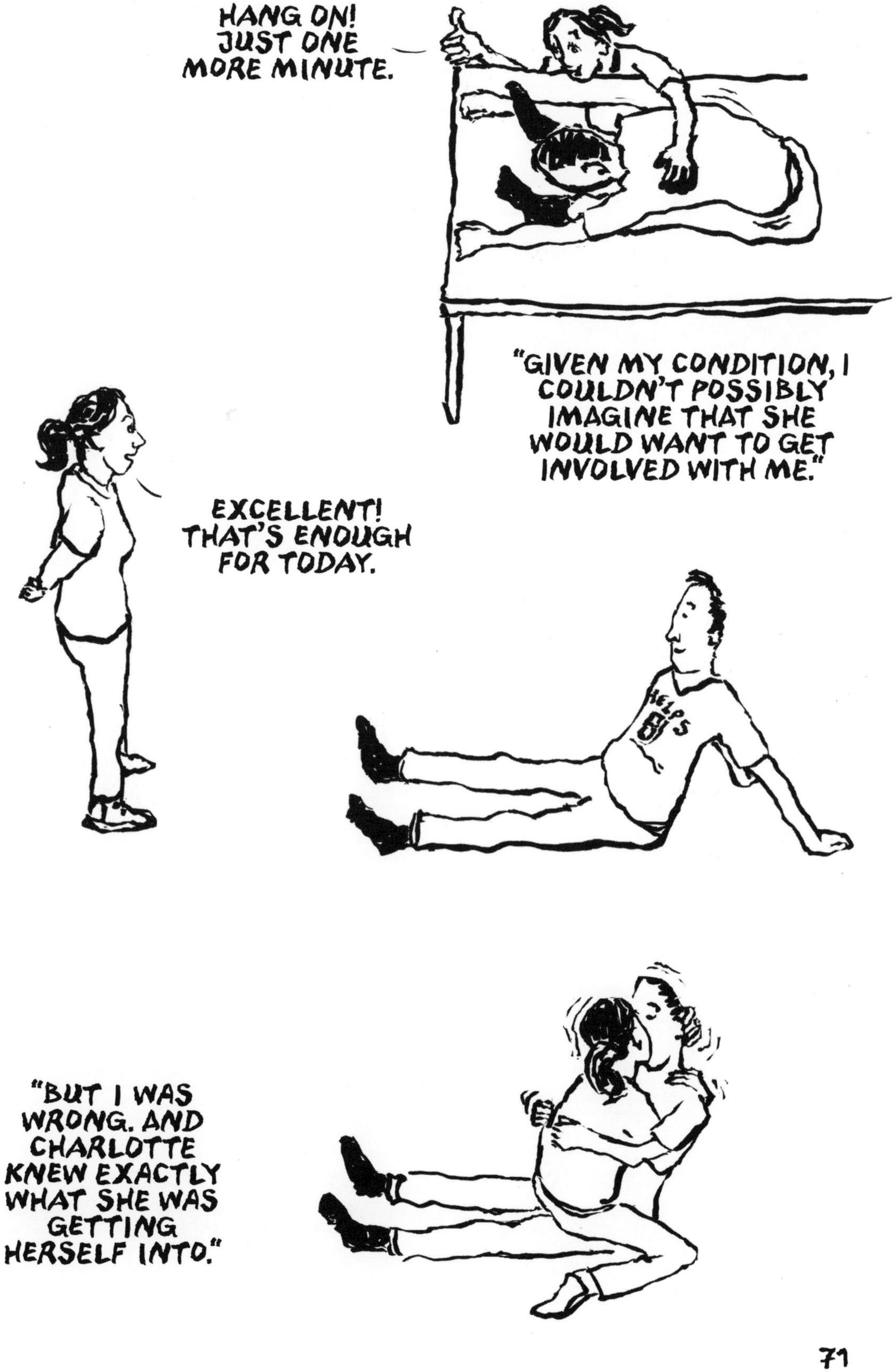
HANG ON! JUST ONE MORE MINUTE.
"GIVEN MY CONDITION, I COULDN'T POSSIBLY IMAGINE THAT SHE WOULD WANT TO GET INVOLVED WITH ME."
EXCELLENT! THAT'S ENOUGH FOR TODAY.
"BUT I WAS WRONG. AND CHARLOTTE KNEW EXACTLY WHAT SHE WAS GETTING HERSELF INTO."

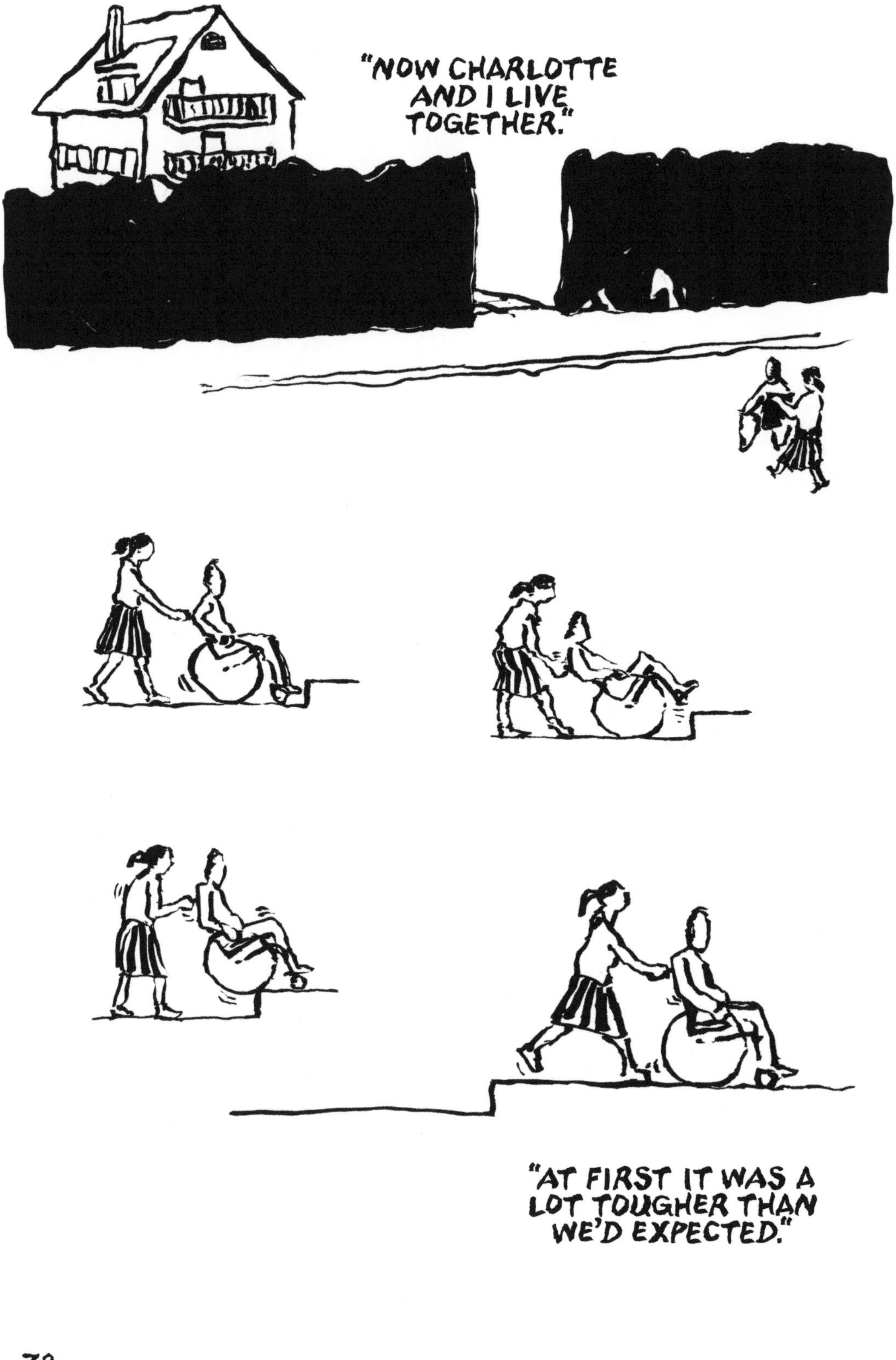
"NOW CHARLOTTE AND I LIVE TOGETHER."
"AT FIRST IT WAS A LOT TOUGHER THAN WE'D EXPECTED."

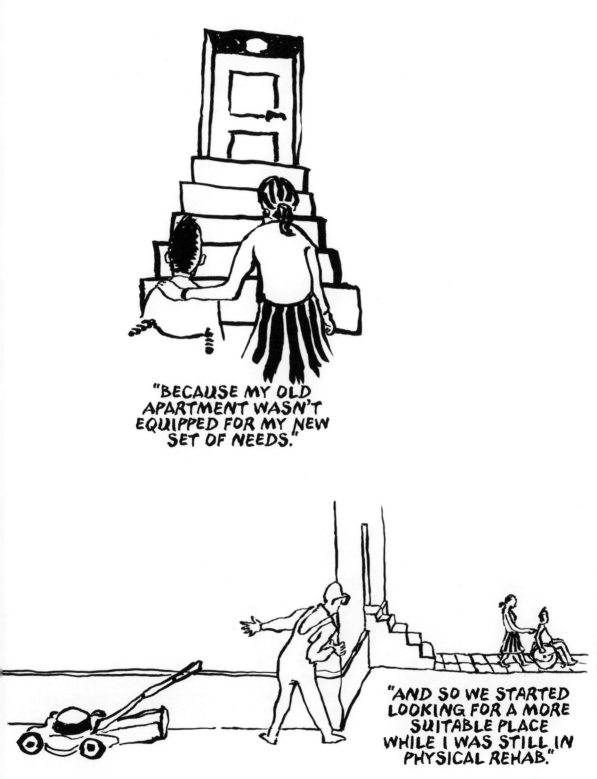

"BECAUSE MY OLD APARTMENT WASN'T EQUIPPED FOR MY NEW SET OF NEEDS."

"AND SO WE STARTED LOOKING FOR A MORE SUITABLE PLACE WHILE I WAS STILL IN PHYSICAL REHAB."

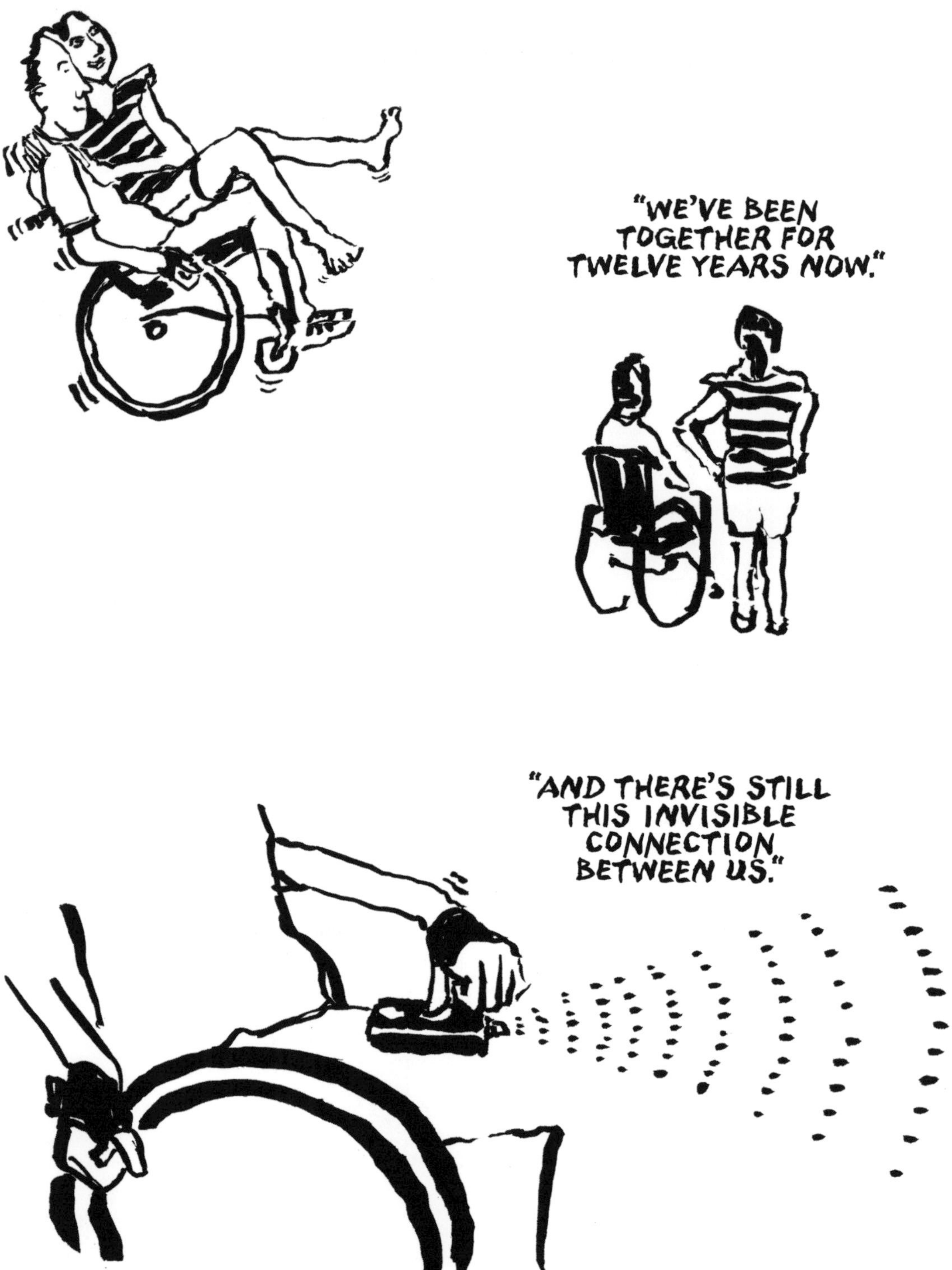
"WE'VE BEEN TOGETHER FOR TWELVE YEARS NOW."
"AND THERE'S STILL THIS INVISIBLE CONNECTION BETWEEN US."

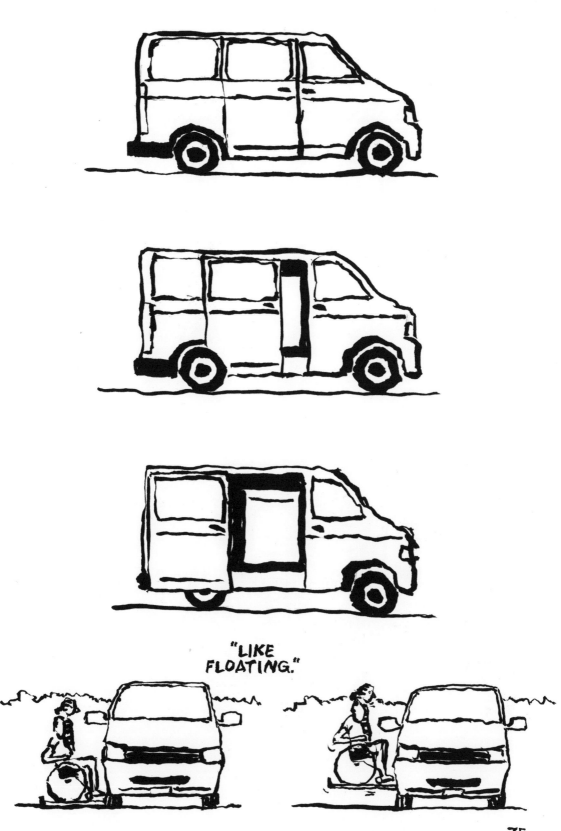

"LIKE
FLOATING."

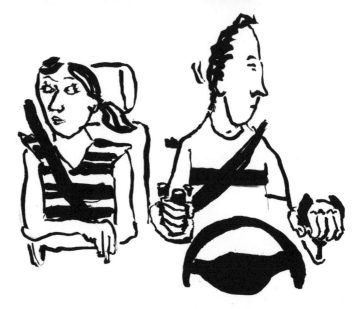

"LOCK THE WHEELCHAIR, HANDS ON THE WHEEL, QUICK CHECK IN THE MIRROR."

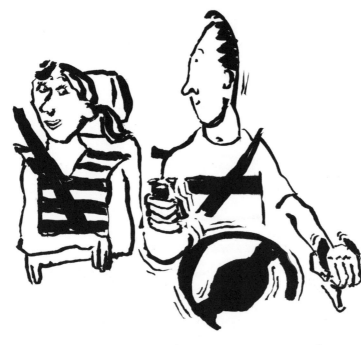

"AND OFF WE GO!"

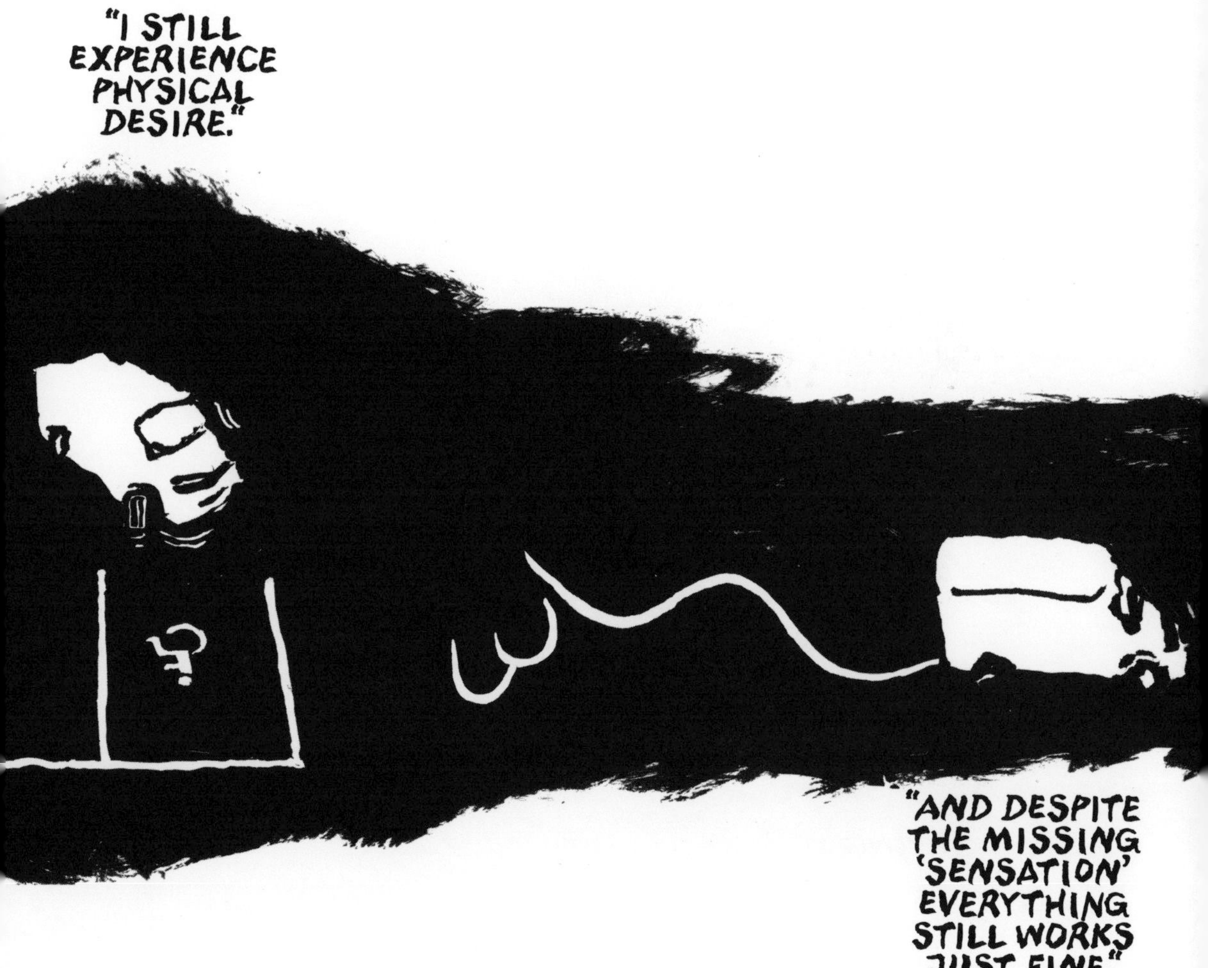
"I STILL EXPERIENCE PHYSICAL DESIRE."
"AND DESPITE THE MISSING 'SENSATION' EVERYTHING STILL WORKS JUST FINE."

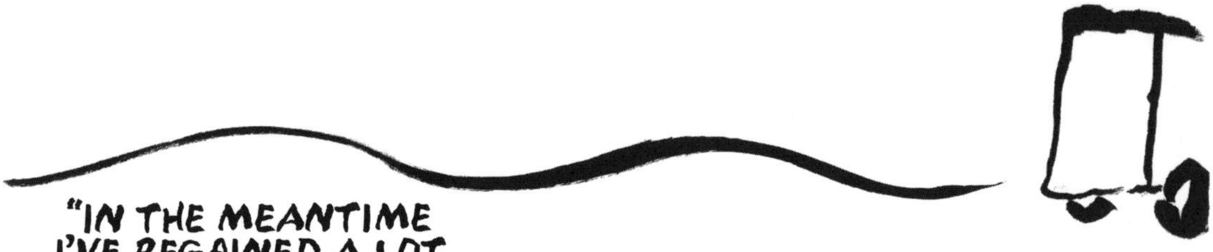

"IN THE MEANTIME I'VE REGAINED A LOT OF FREEDOM AND INDEPENDENCE."

"I'VE STOPPED..."

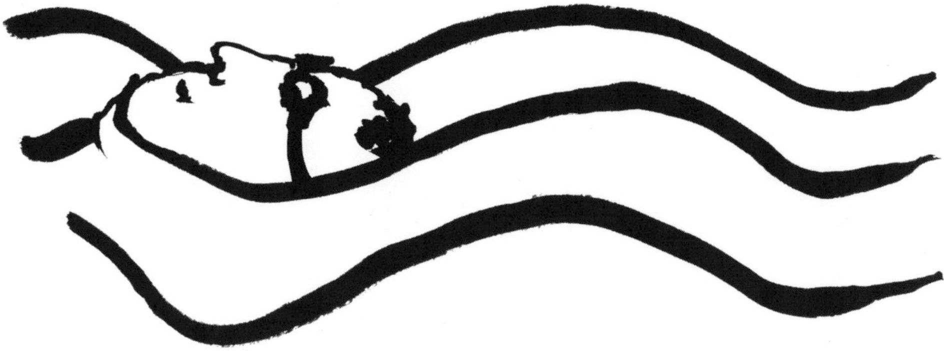

"FIGHTING IT."

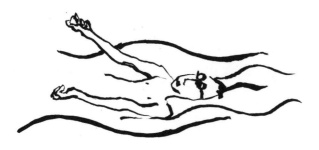

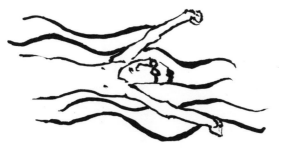

"AND I'VE LEARNED..."

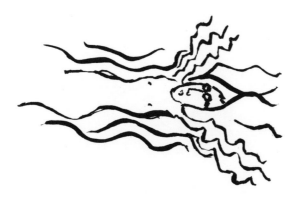

"TO JUST GO WITH THE FLOW."

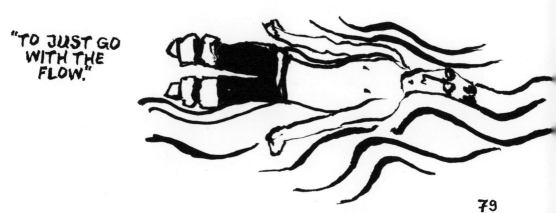

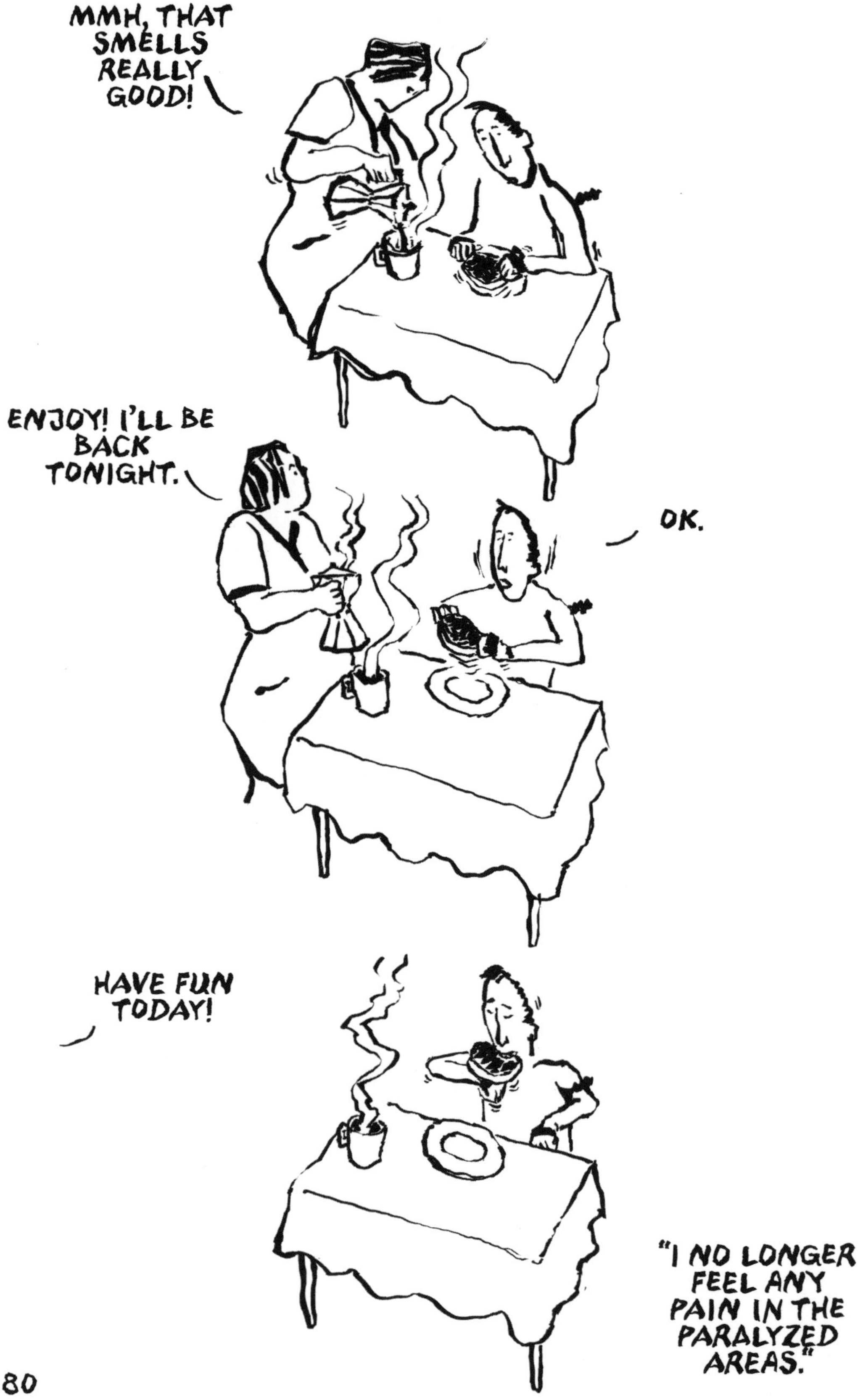
MMH, THAT SMELLS REALLY GOOD!
ENJOY! I'LL BE BACK TONIGHT.
OK.
HAVE FUN TODAY!
"I NO LONGER FEEL ANY PAIN IN THE PARALYZED AREAS."

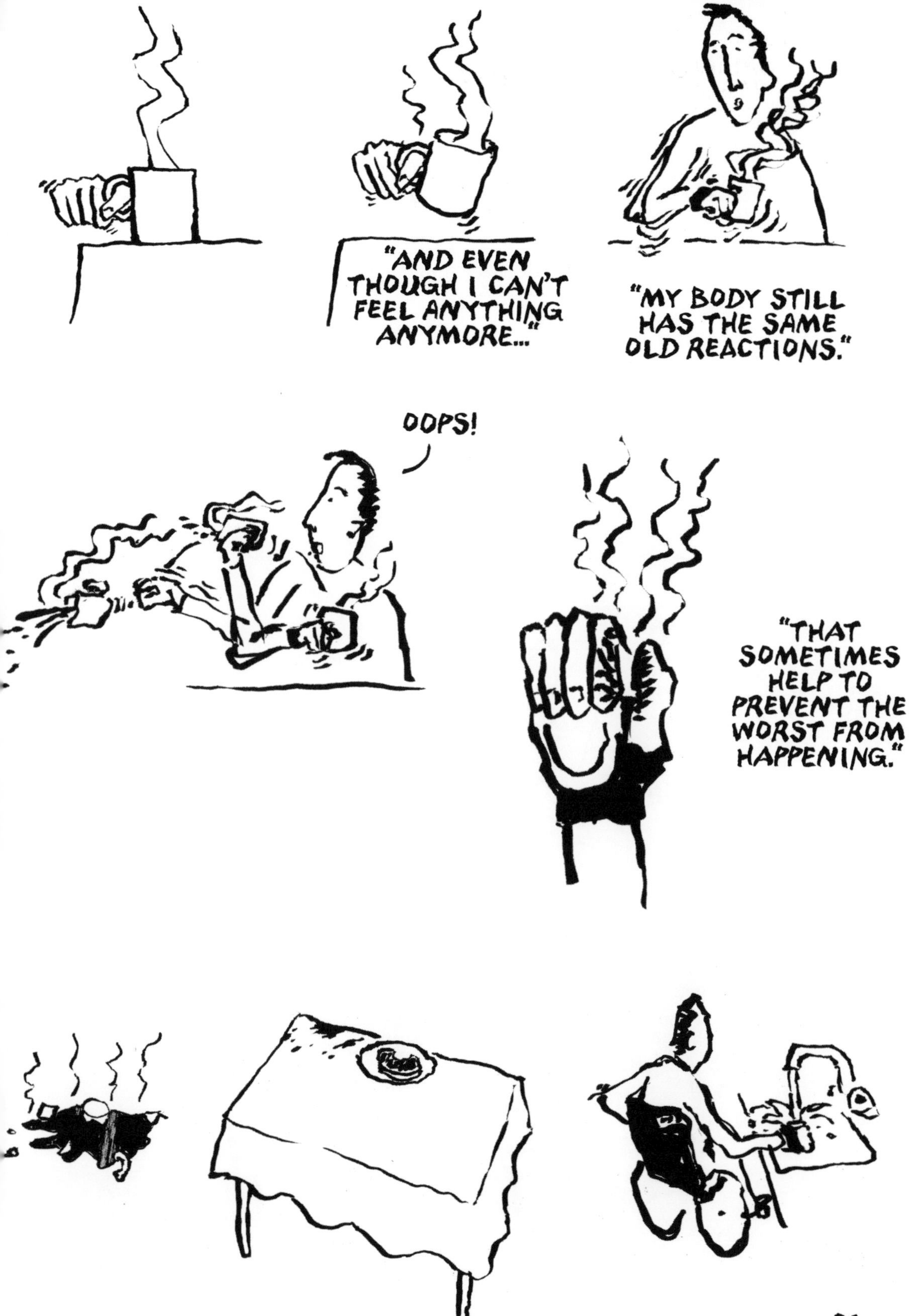
"AND EVEN THOUGH I CAN'T FEEL ANYTHING ANYMORE..."
"MY BODY STILL HAS THE SAME OLD REACTIONS."
OOPS!
"THAT SOMETIMES HELP TO PREVENT THE WORST FROM HAPPENING."

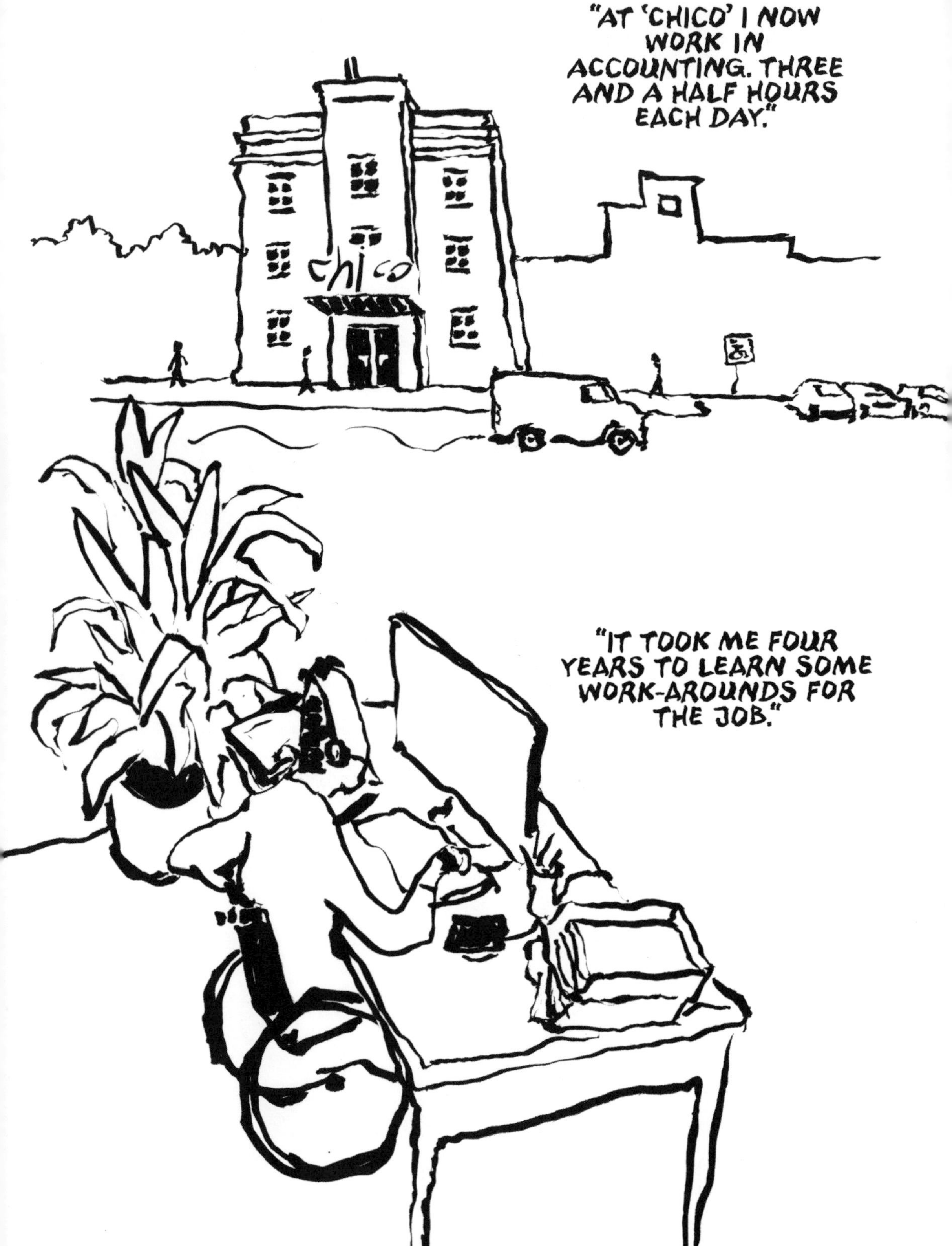
"AT 'CHICO' I NOW WORK IN ACCOUNTING. THREE AND A HALF HOURS EACH DAY."
"IT TOOK ME FOUR YEARS TO LEARN SOME WORK-AROUNDS FOR THE JOB."

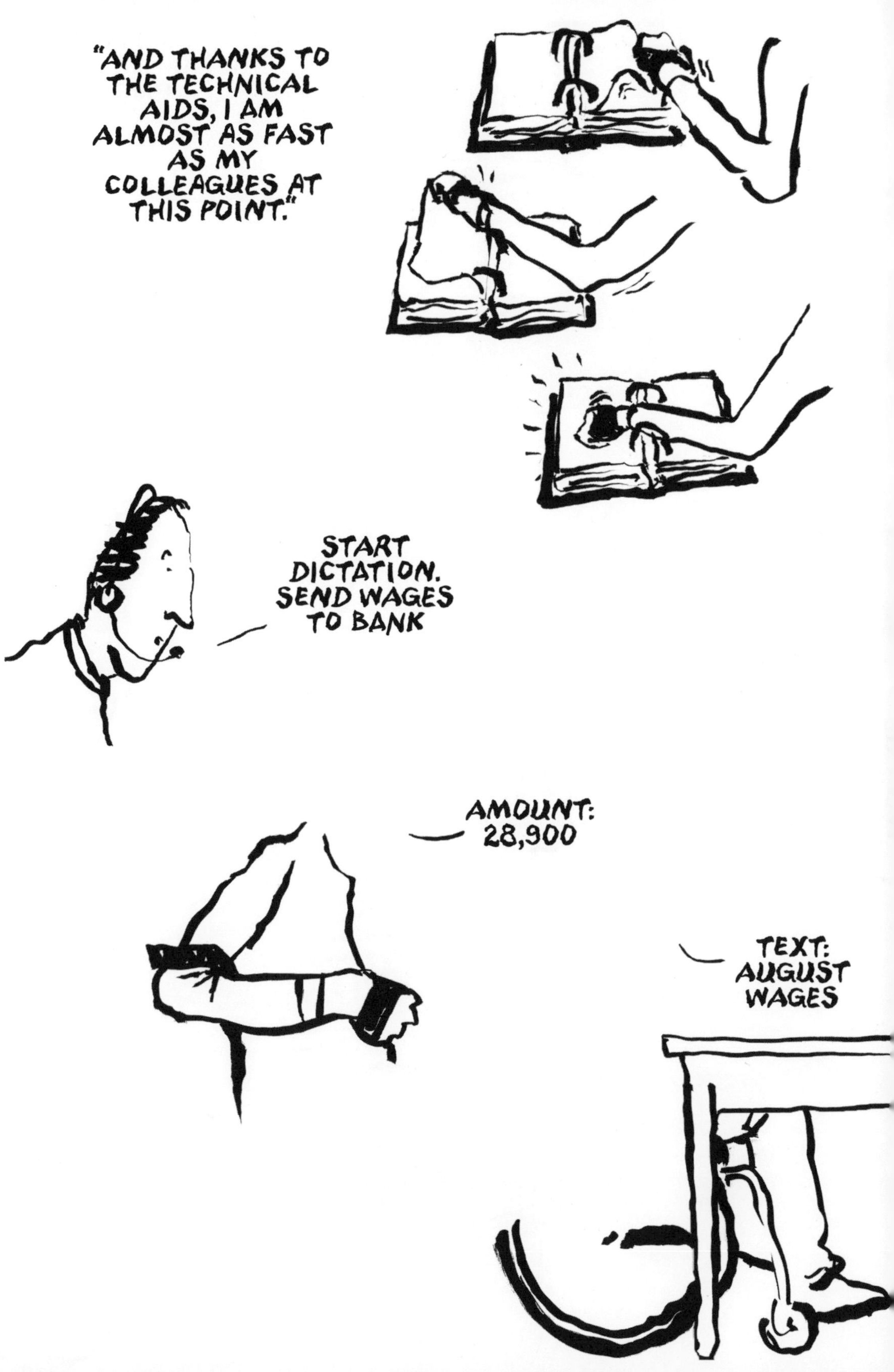
"AND THANKS TO THE TECHNICAL AIDS, I AM ALMOST AS FAST AS MY COLLEAGUES AT THIS POINT."
START DICTATION. SEND WAGES TO BANK
AMOUNT: 28,900
TEXT: AUGUST WAGES

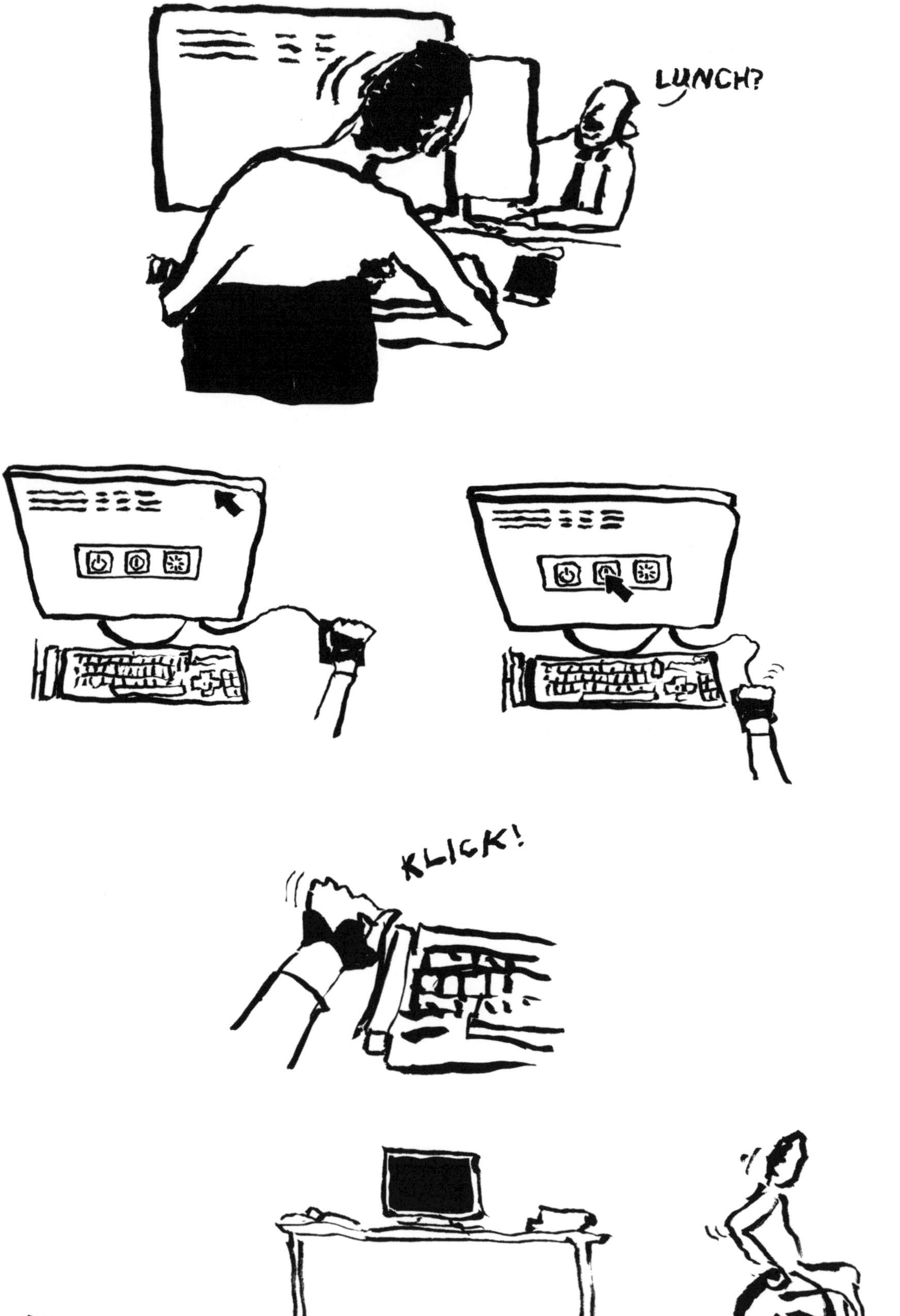
LUNCH?
KLICK!

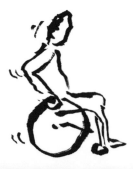

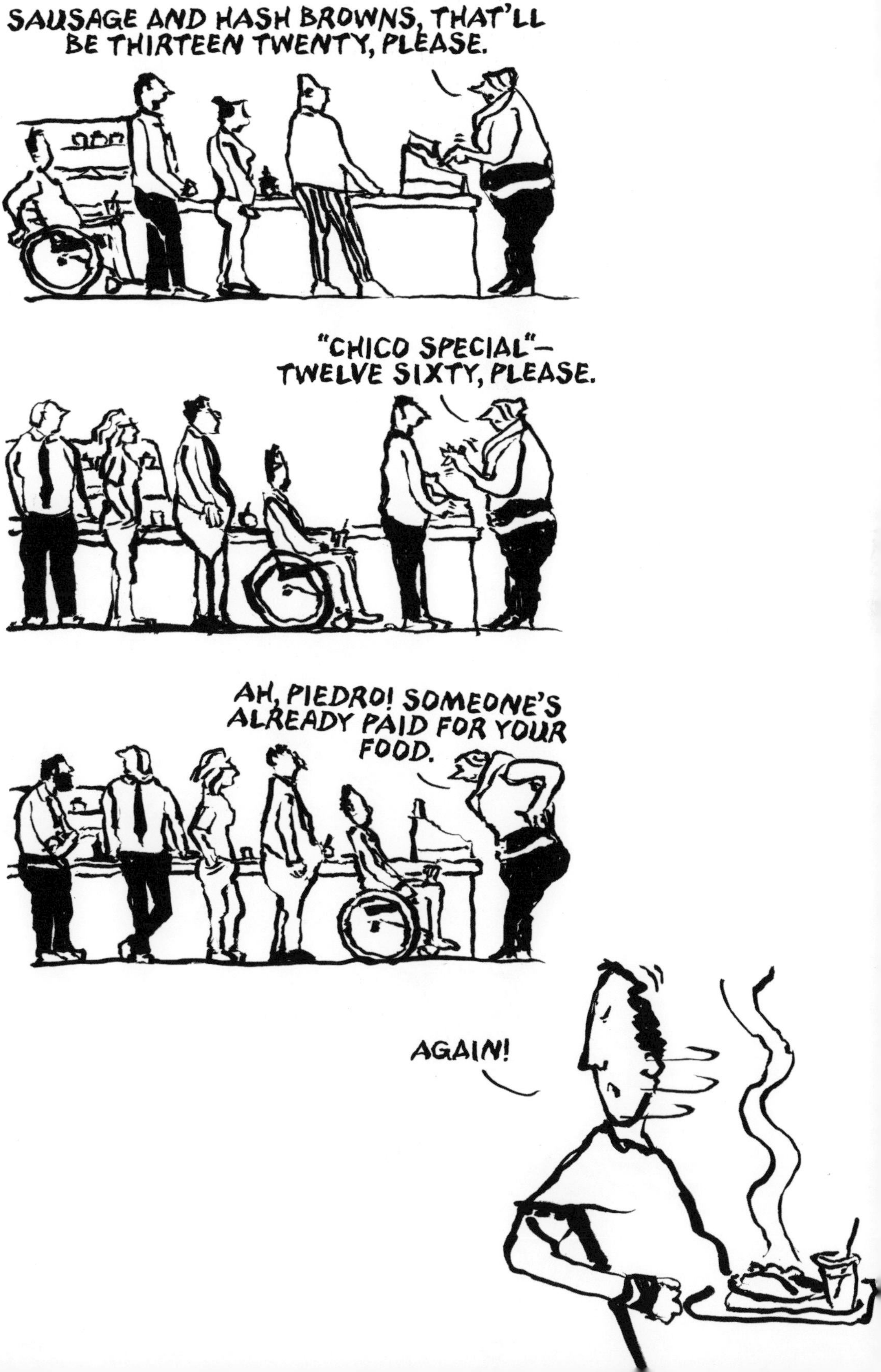
SAUSAGE AND HASH BROWNS, THAT'LL BE THIRTEEN TWENTY, PLEASE.
"CHICO SPECIAL"— TWELVE SIXTY, PLEASE.
AH, PIEDRO! SOMEONE'S ALREADY PAID FOR YOUR FOOD.
AGAIN!

"THE FIRST STAGE OF REHAB LASTED THE ENTIRE WINTER."

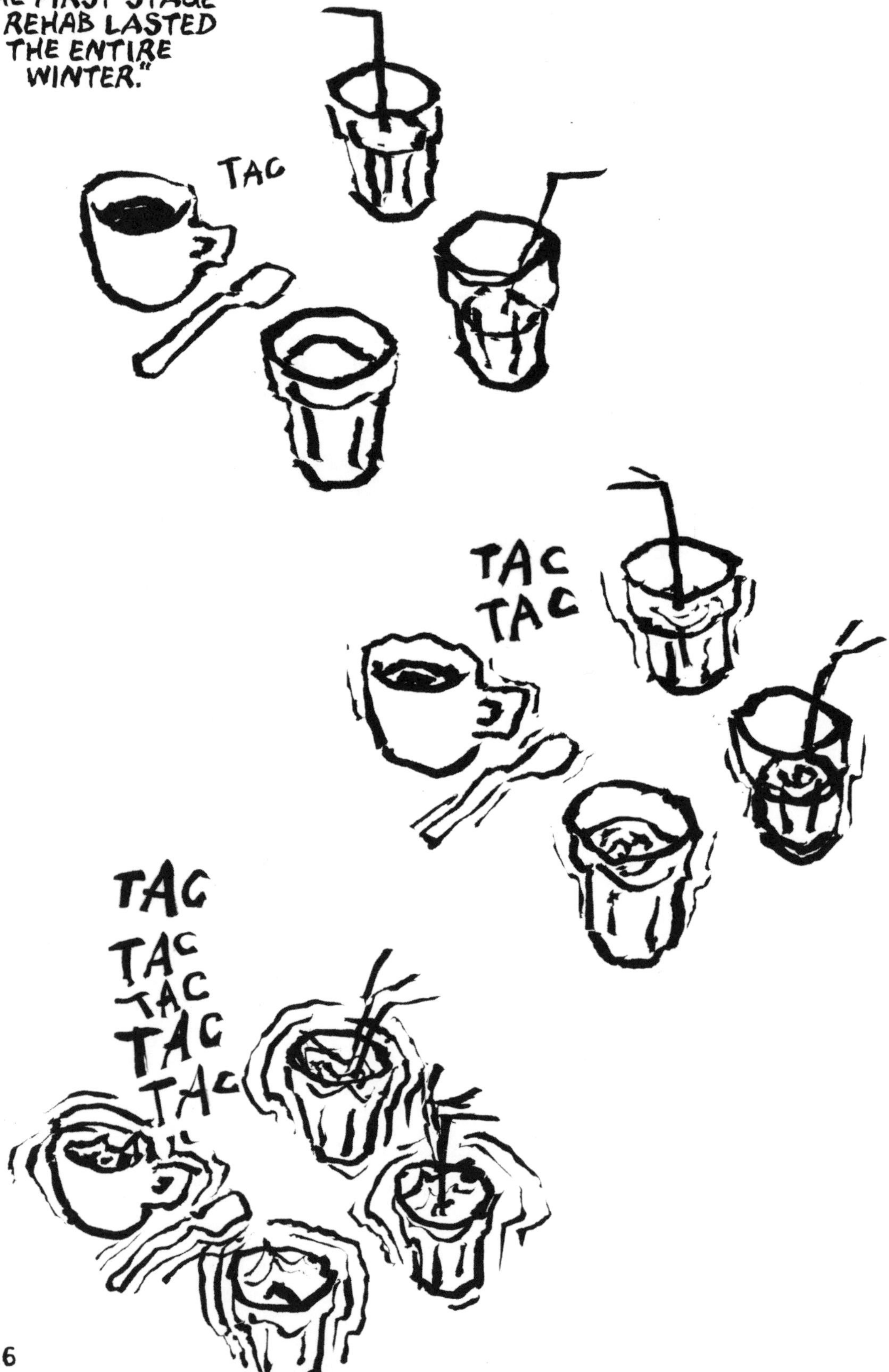
TAC
TAC
TAC
TAG
TAC
TAC
TAC
TAC

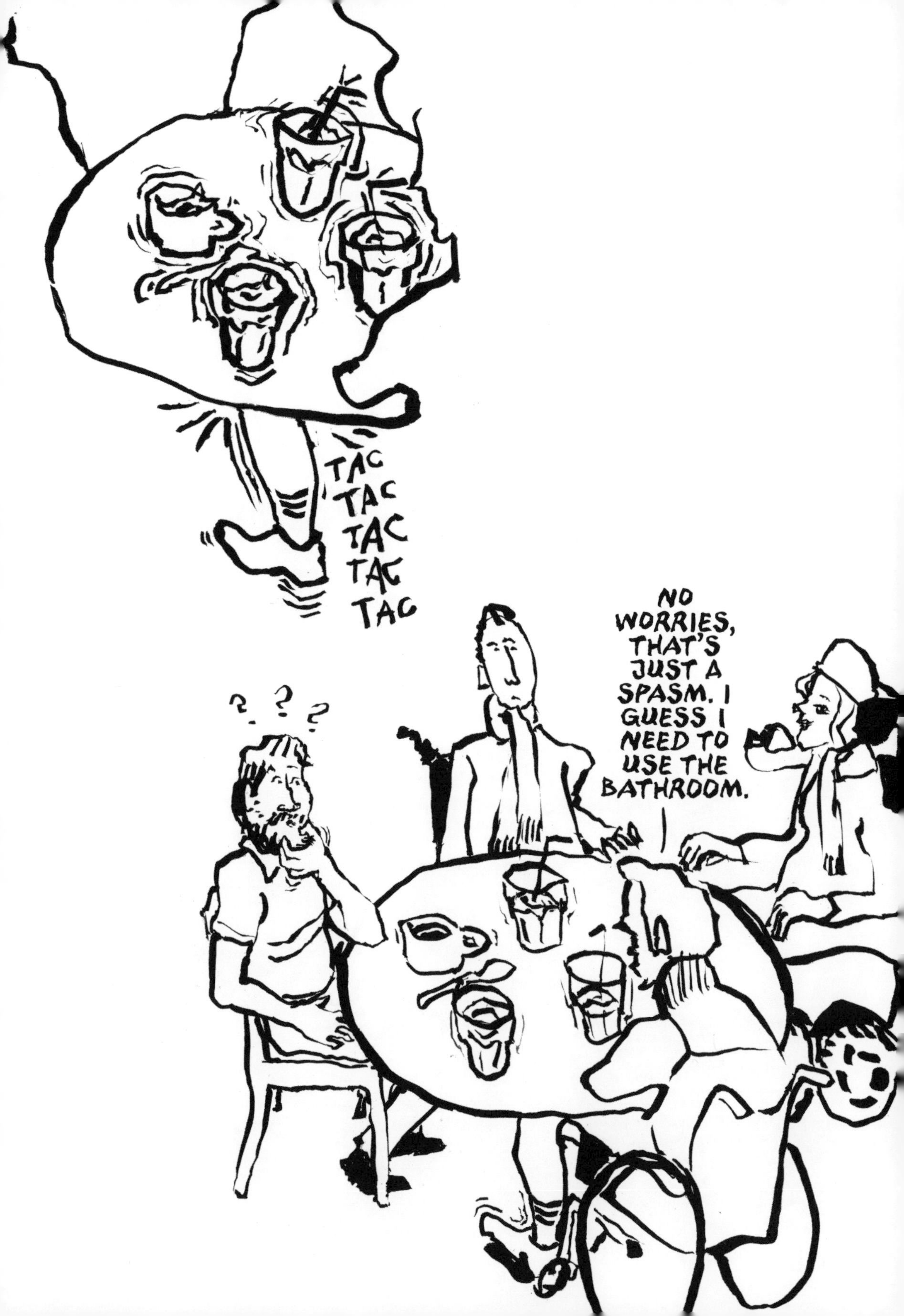
TAC
TAC
TAC
TAC
TAC
? ? ?
NO WORRIES, THAT'S JUST A SPASM. I GUESS I NEED TO USE THE BATHROOM.

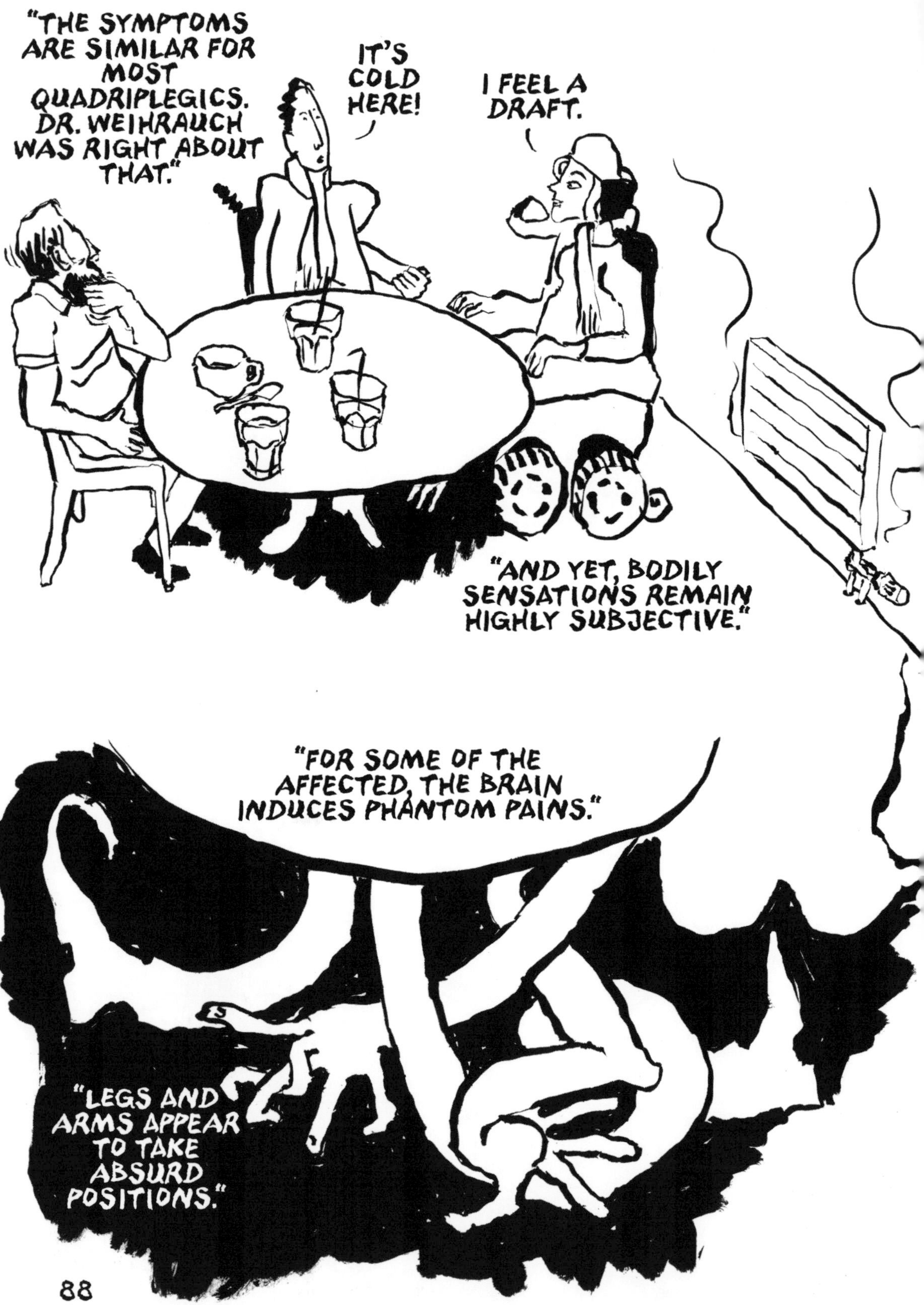
"THE SYMPTOMS ARE SIMILAR FOR MOST QUADRIPLEGICS. DR. WEIHRAUCH WAS RIGHT ABOUT THAT."
IT'S COLD HERE!
I FEEL A DRAFT.
"AND YET, BODILY SENSATIONS REMAIN HIGHLY SUBJECTIVE."
"FOR SOME OF THE AFFECTED, THE BRAIN INDUCES PHANTOM PAINS."
"LEGS AND ARMS APPEAR TO TAKE ABSURD POSITIONS."

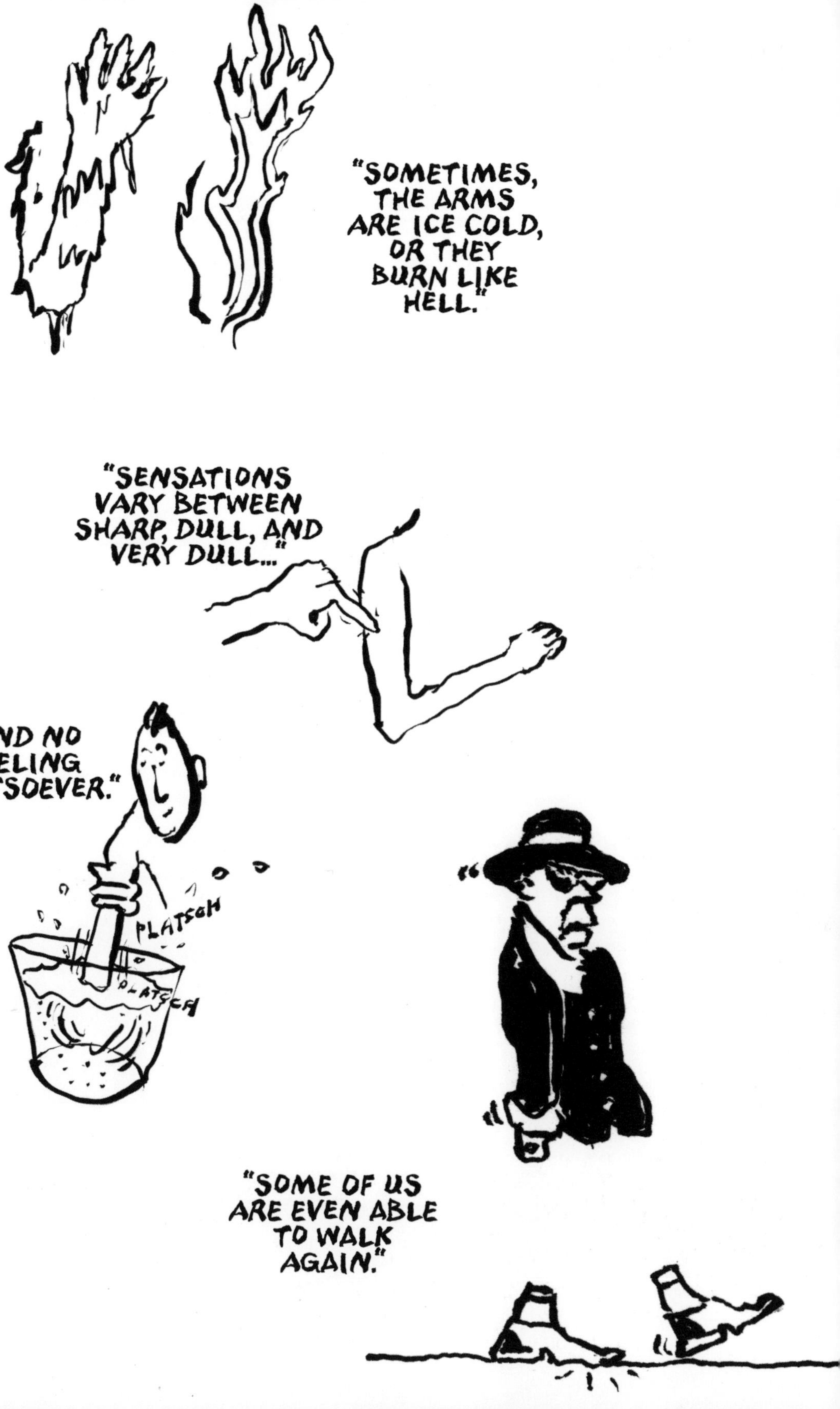
"SOMETIMES, THE ARMS ARE ICE COLD, OR THEY BURN LIKE HELL."
"SENSATIONS VARY BETWEEN SHARP, DULL, AND VERY DULL..."
"AND NO FEELING WHATSOEVER."
PLATSCH
PLATSCH
"SOME OF US ARE EVEN ABLE TO WALK AGAIN."

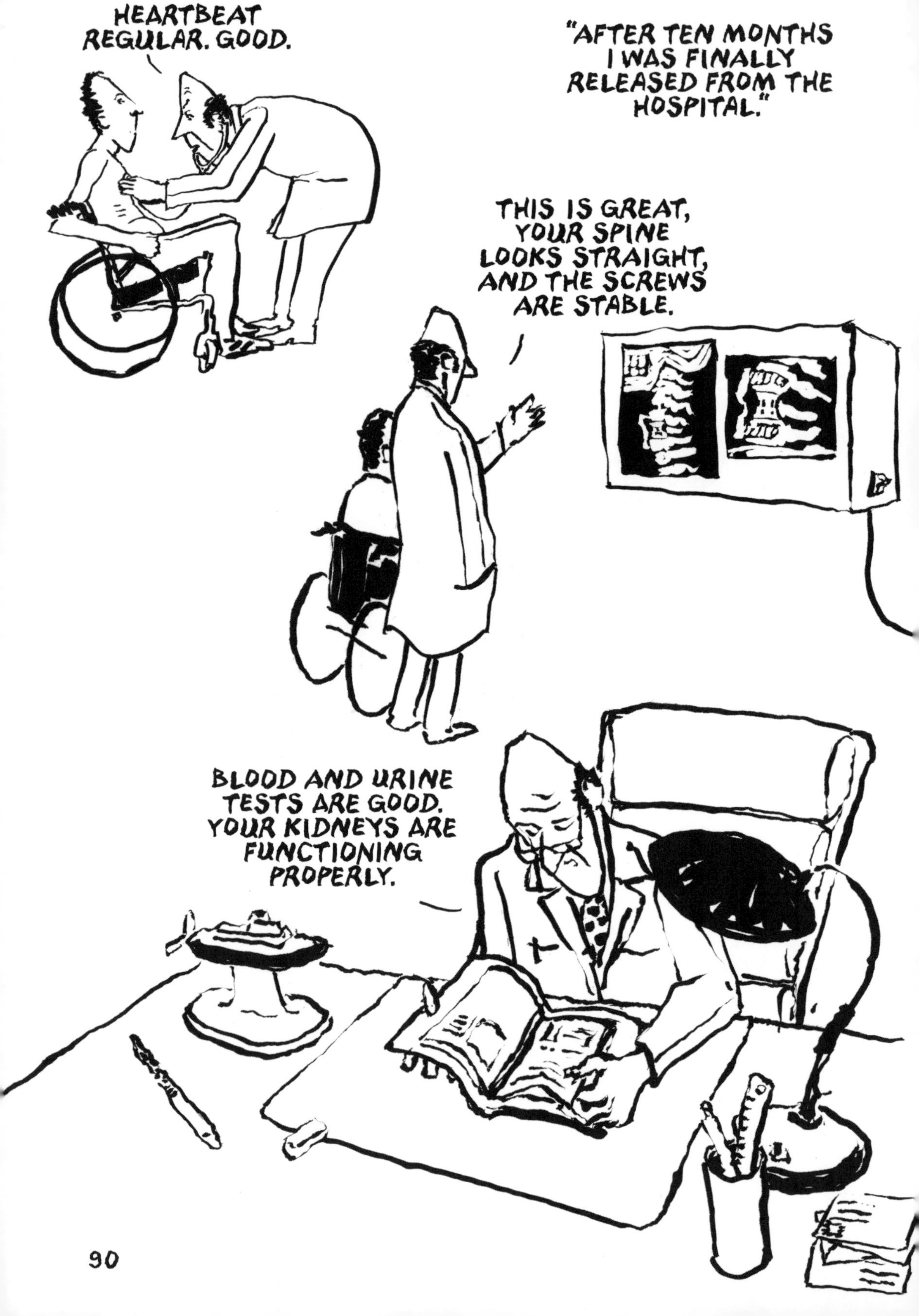
HEARTBEAT REGULAR. GOOD.
"AFTER TEN MONTHS I WAS FINALLY RELEASED FROM THE HOSPITAL."
THIS IS GREAT, YOUR SPINE LOOKS STRAIGHT, AND THE SCREWS ARE STABLE.
BLOOD AND URINE TESTS ARE GOOD. YOUR KIDNEYS ARE FUNCTIONING PROPERLY.

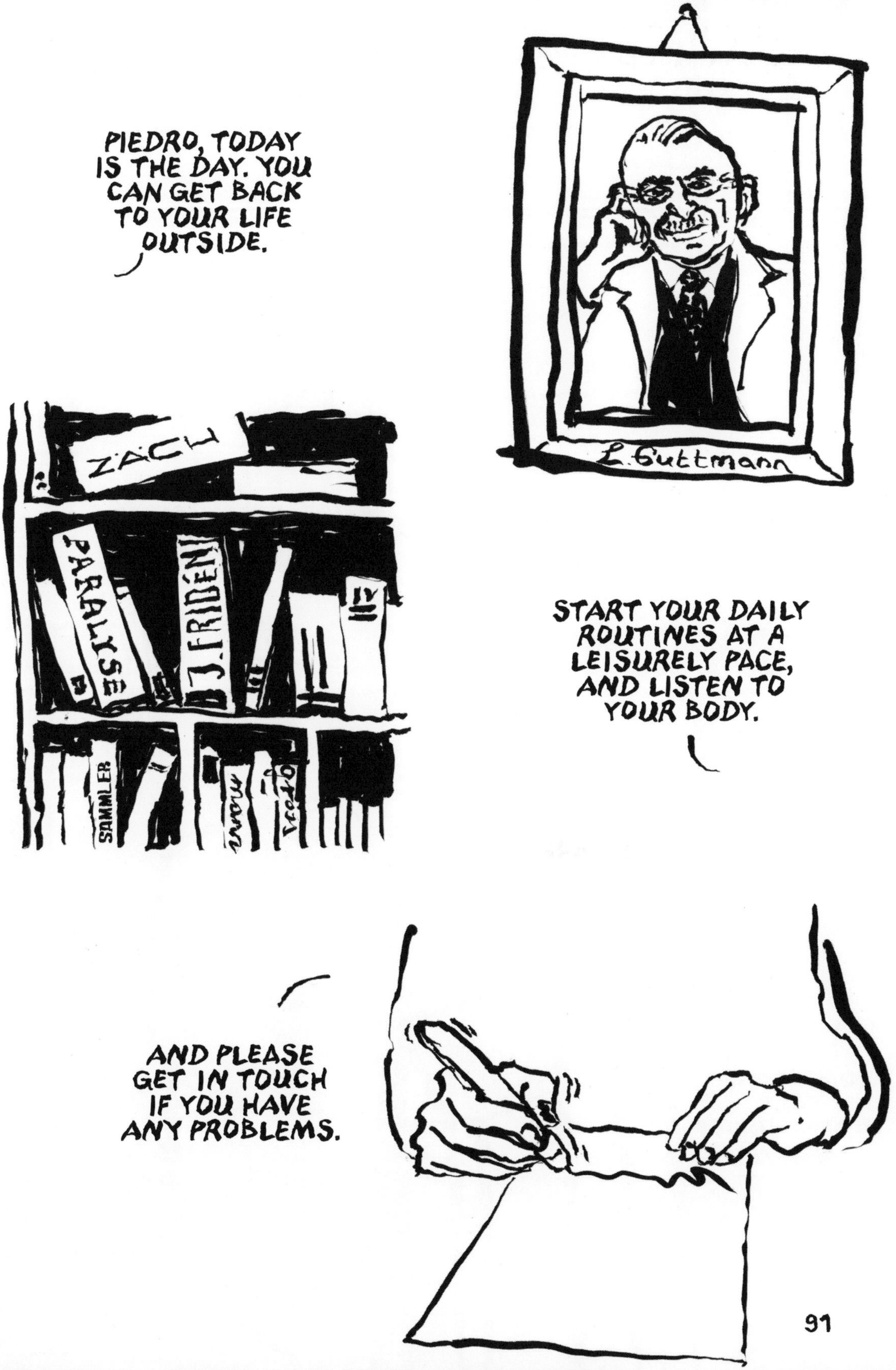
PIEDRO, TODAY IS THE DAY. YOU CAN GET BACK TO YOUR LIFE OUTSIDE.
L. Guttmann
ZACH
PARALYSE
J. FRIDÉN
SAMMLER
START YOUR DAILY ROUTINES AT A LEISURELY PACE, AND LISTEN TO YOUR BODY.
AND PLEASE GET IN TOUCH IF YOU HAVE ANY PROBLEMS.

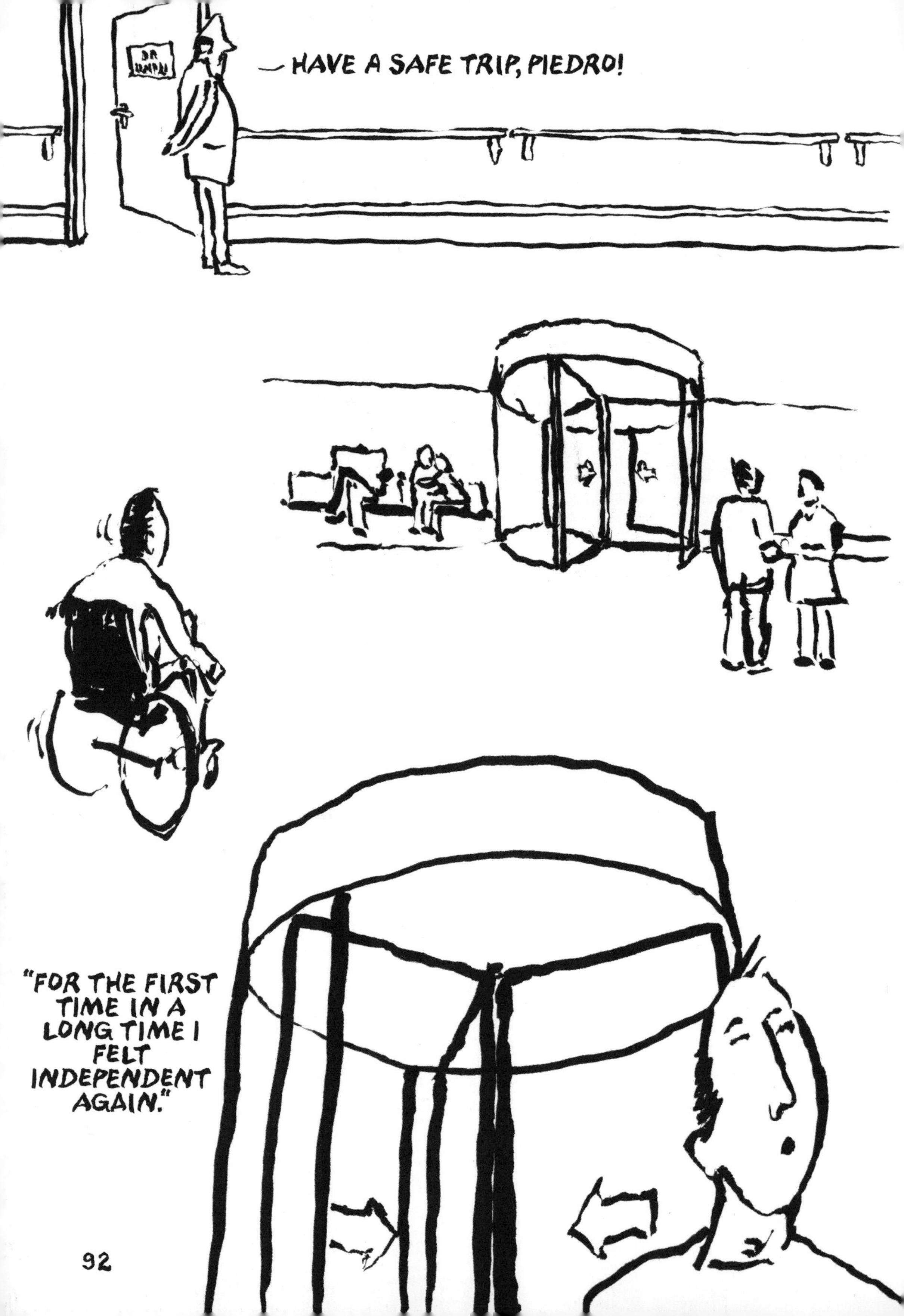
— HAVE A SAFE TRIP, PIEDRO!
"FOR THE FIRST TIME IN A LONG TIME I FELT INDEPENDENT AGAIN."

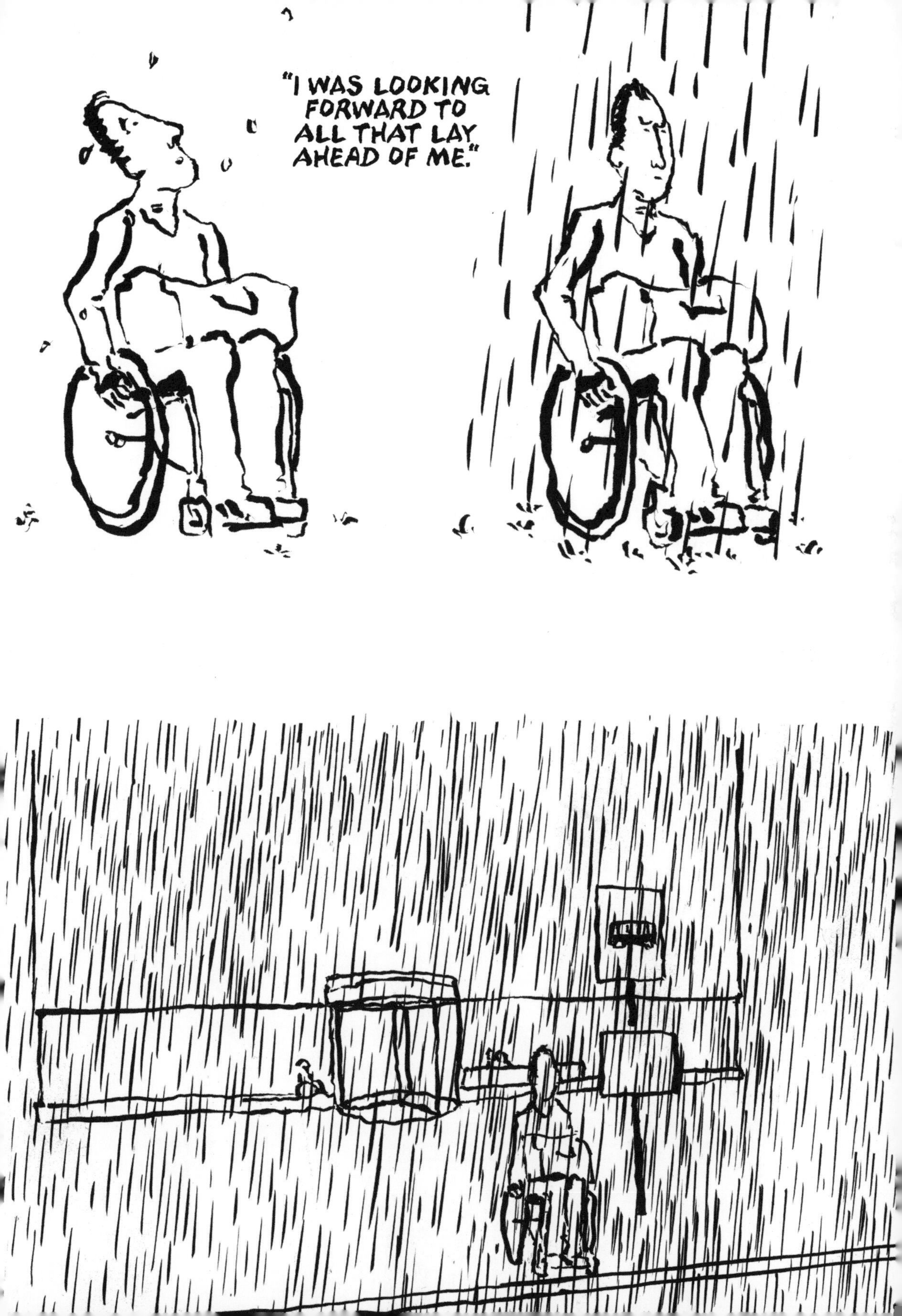
"I WAS LOOKING FORWARD TO ALL THAT LAY AHEAD OF ME."

"I WOULD STILL NEED HELP FROM OTHERS."

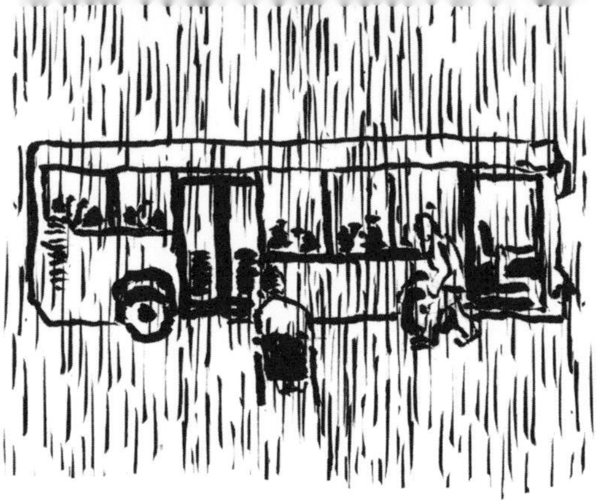

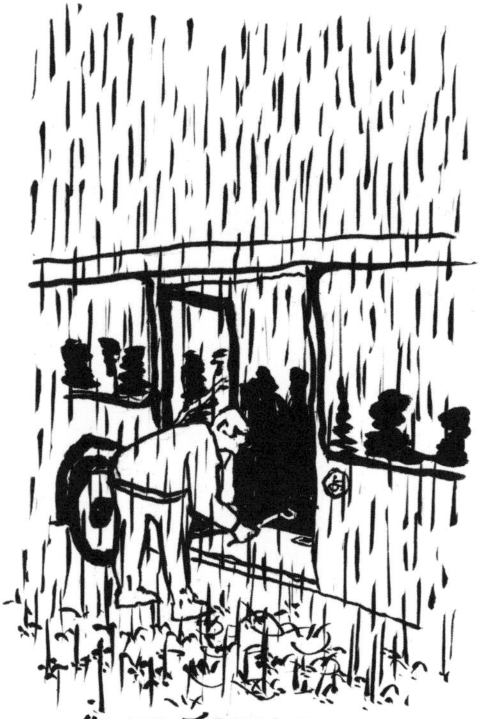

"AND ASKING COMPLETE STRANGERS..."

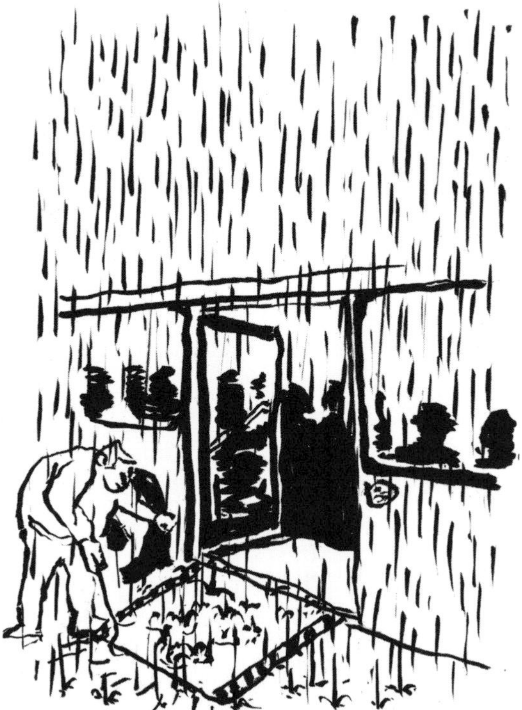

"TO HELP WITH ALL THE LITTLE THINGS I CAN NO LONGER DO ON MY OWN—"

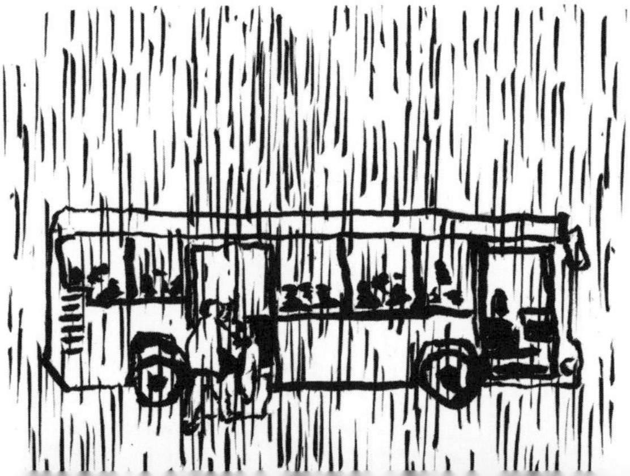

"THAT I WILL NEVER GET USED TO."

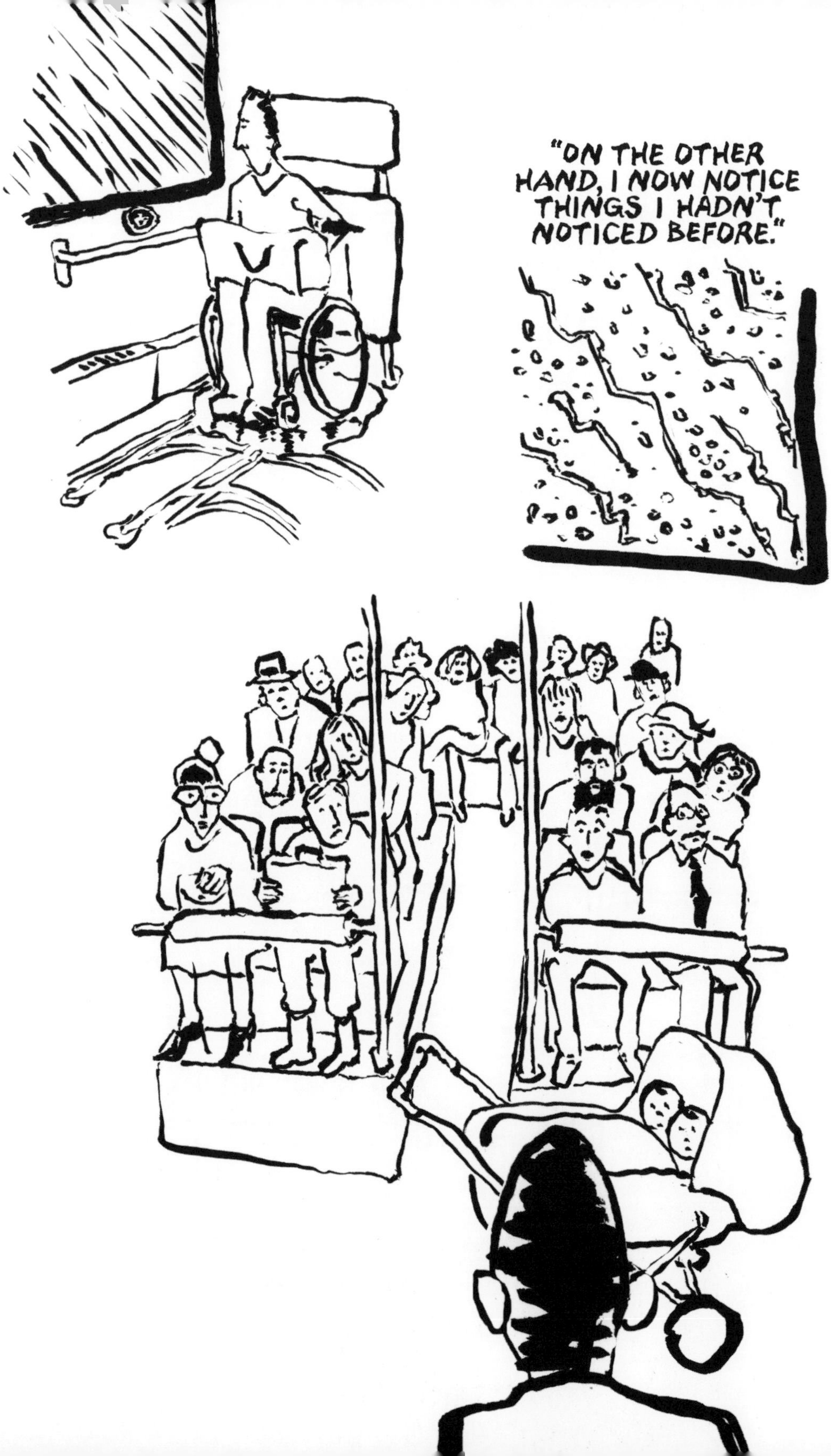
"ON THE OTHER HAND, I NOW NOTICE THINGS I HADN'T NOTICED BEFORE."

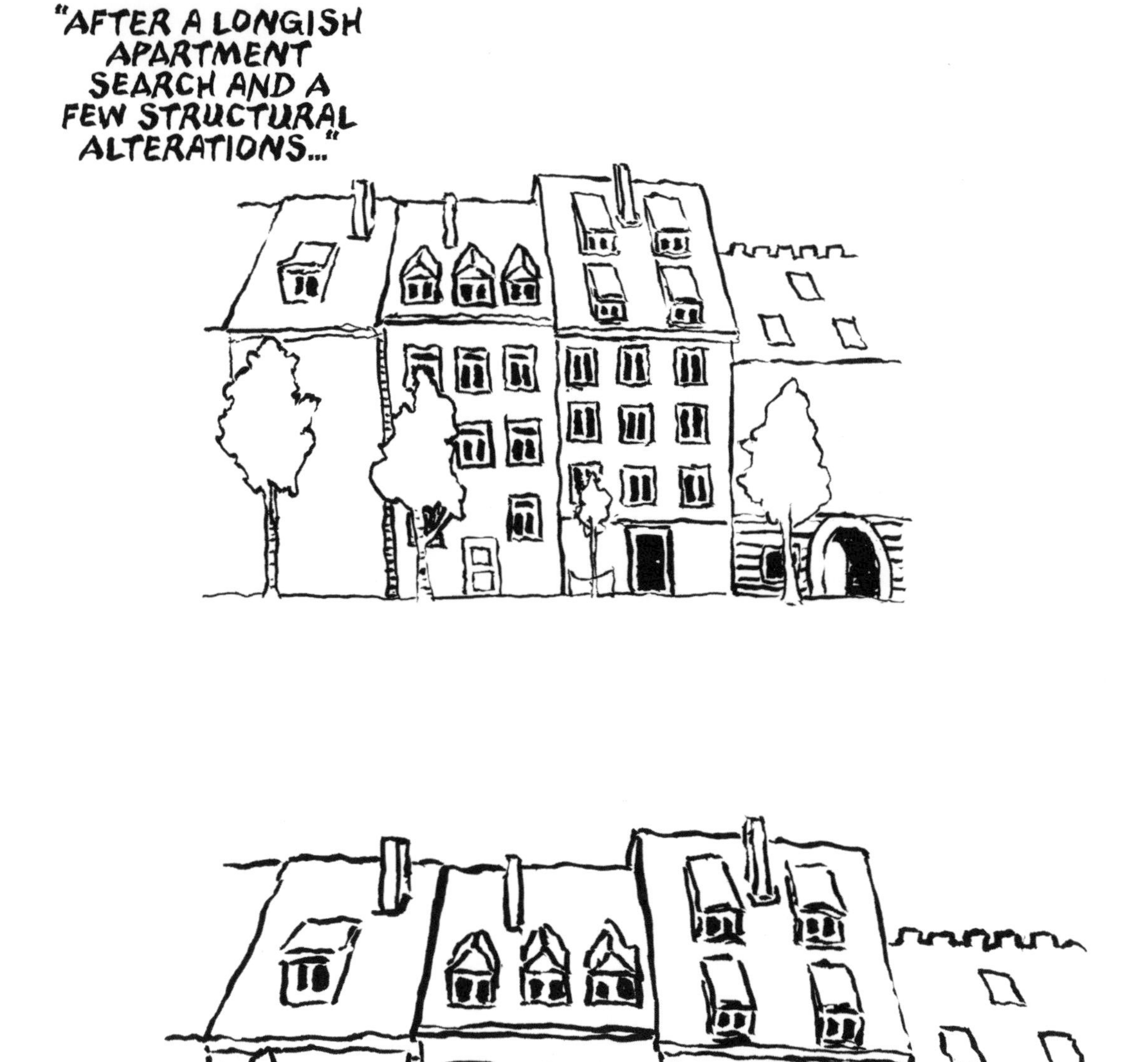
"AFTER A LONGISH APARTMENT SEARCH AND A FEW STRUCTURAL ALTERATIONS..."
"WE COULD FINALLY MOVE INTO OUR NEW HOME."

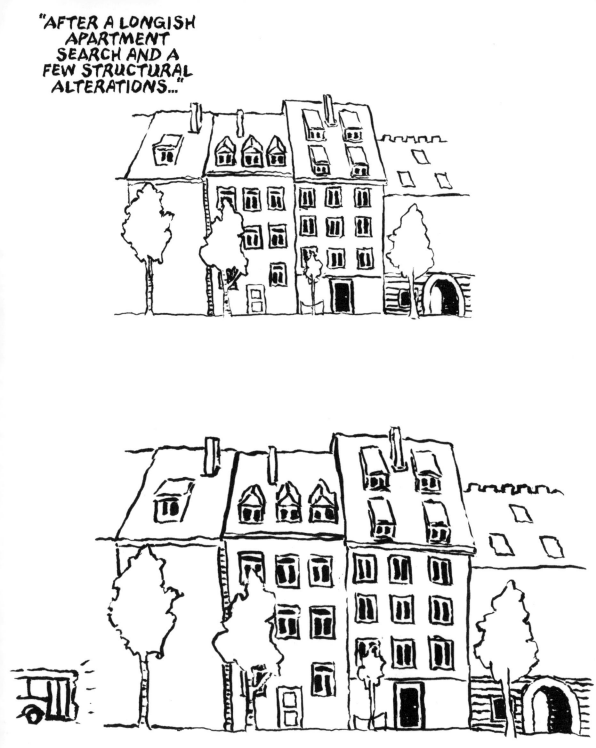

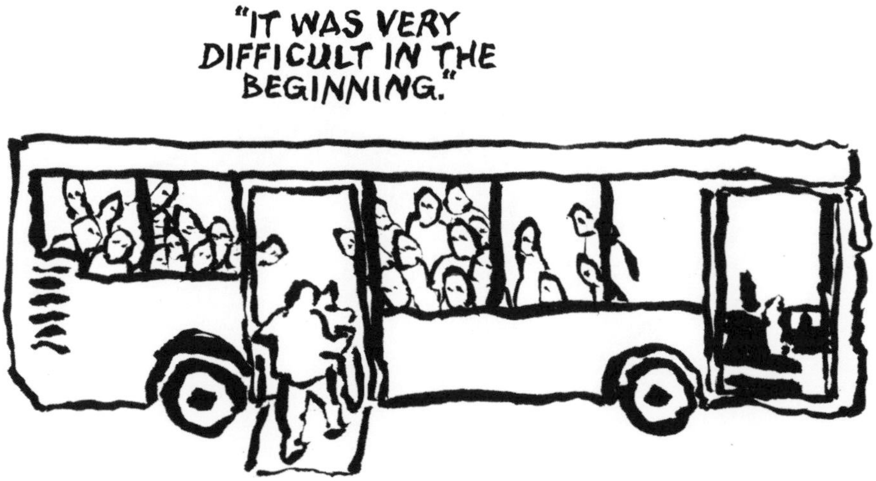
"IT WAS VERY DIFFICULT IN THE BEGINNING."

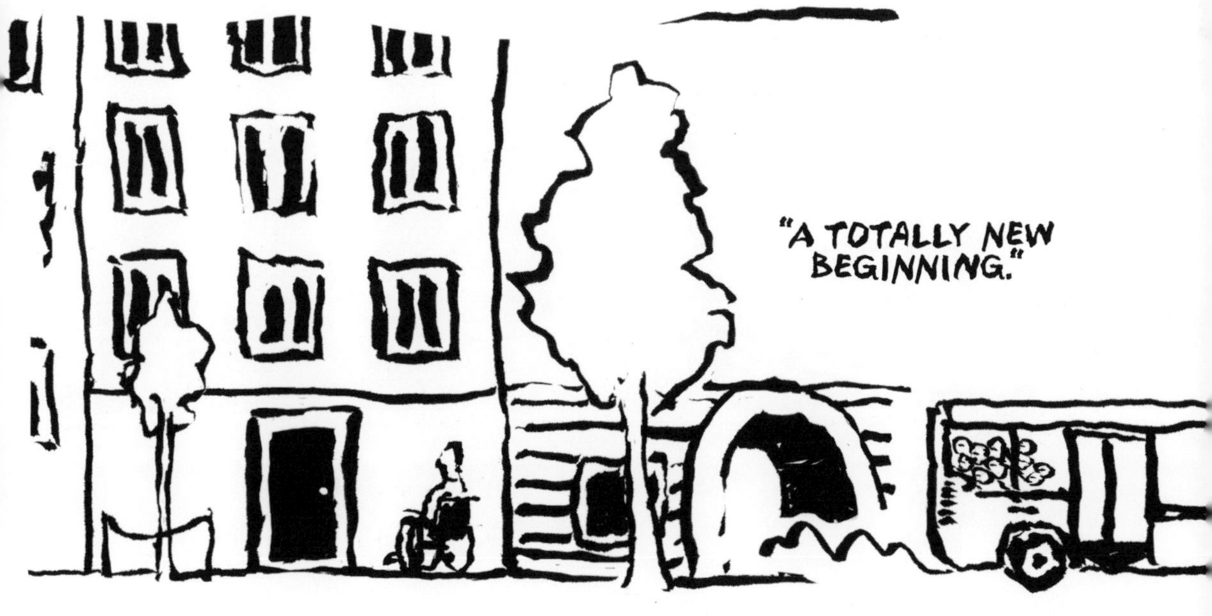
"A TOTALLY NEW BEGINNING."

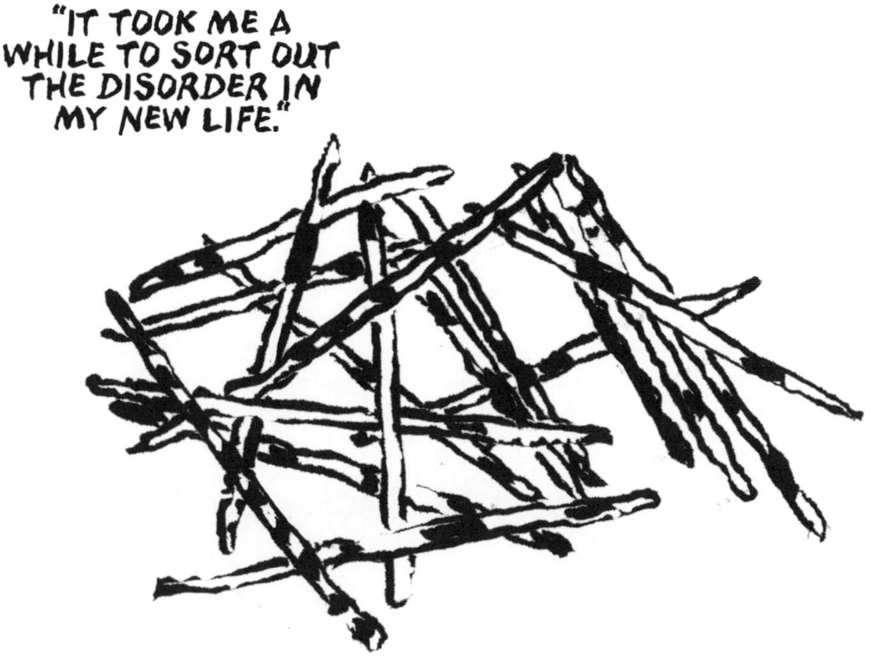
"IT TOOK ME A WHILE TO SORT OUT THE DISORDER IN MY NEW LIFE."

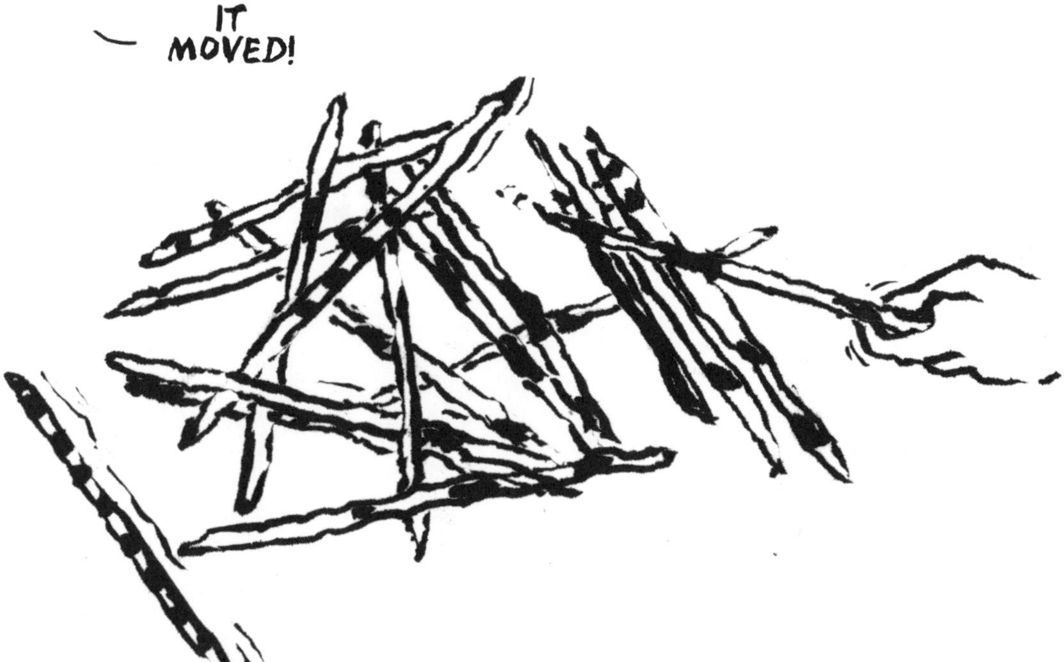
IT MOVED!

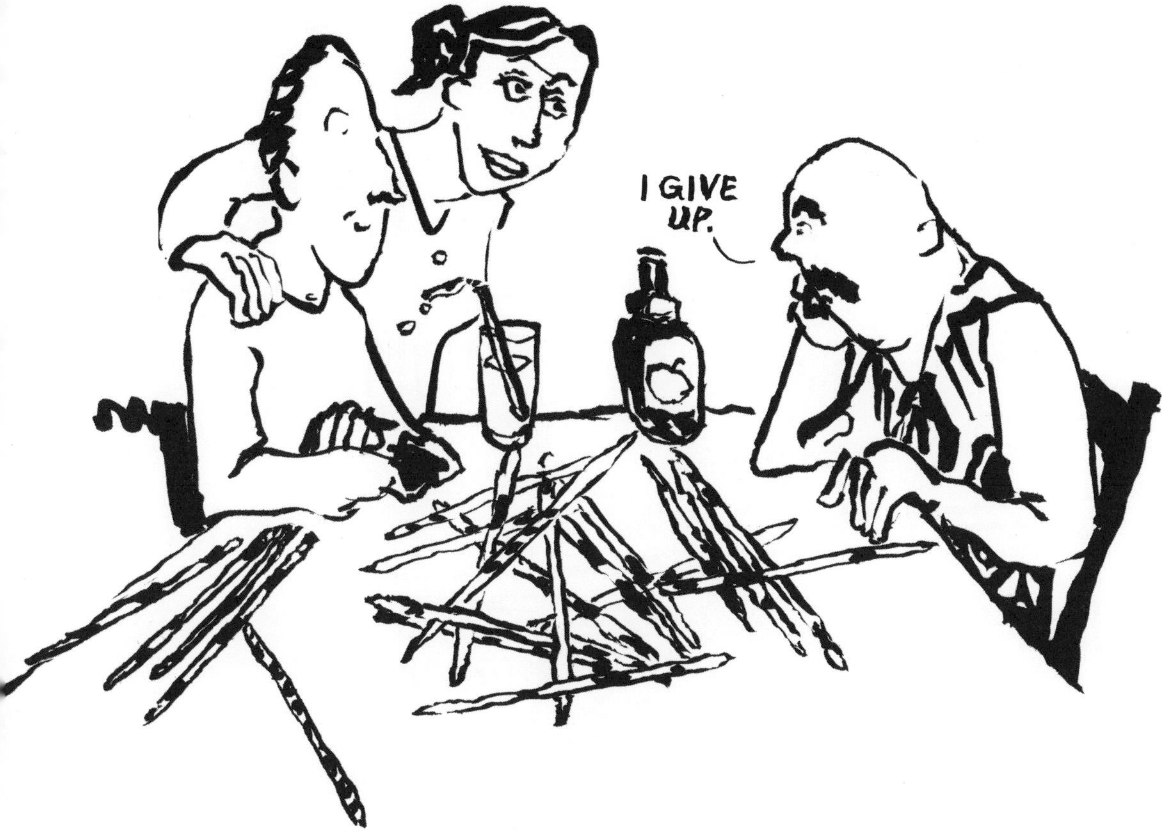
I GIVE UP.

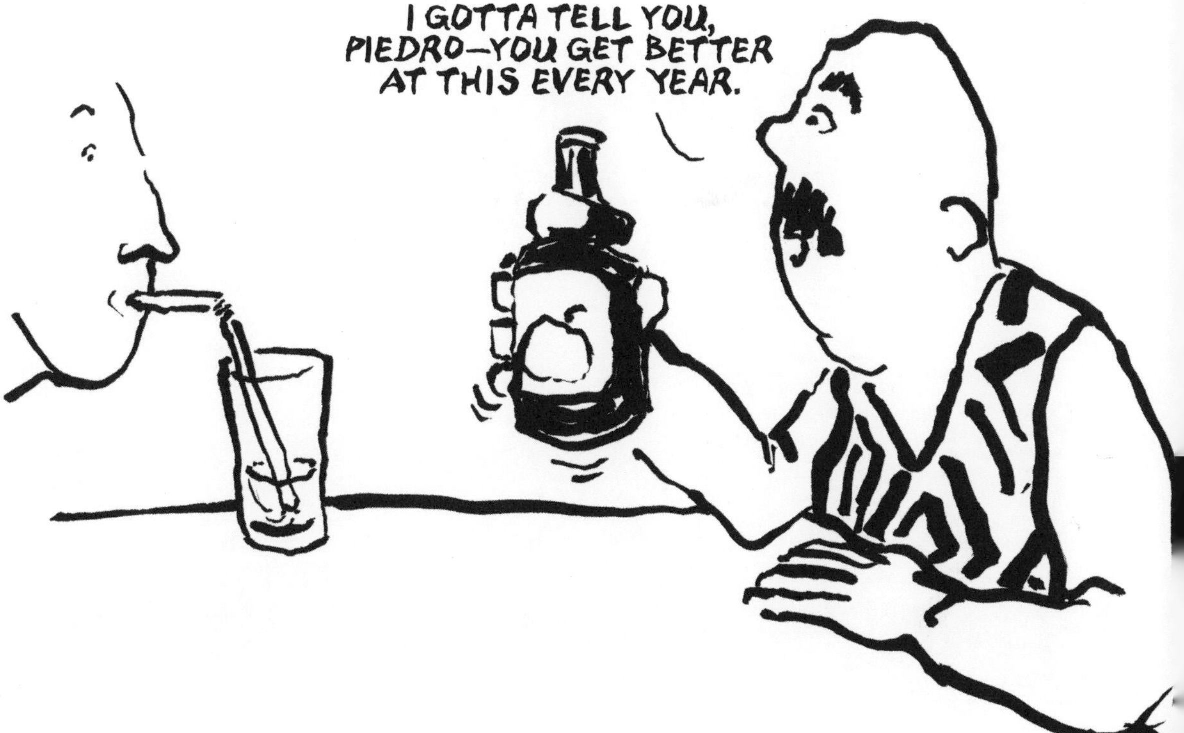
I GOTTA TELL YOU, PIEDRO—YOU GET BETTER AT THIS EVERY YEAR.

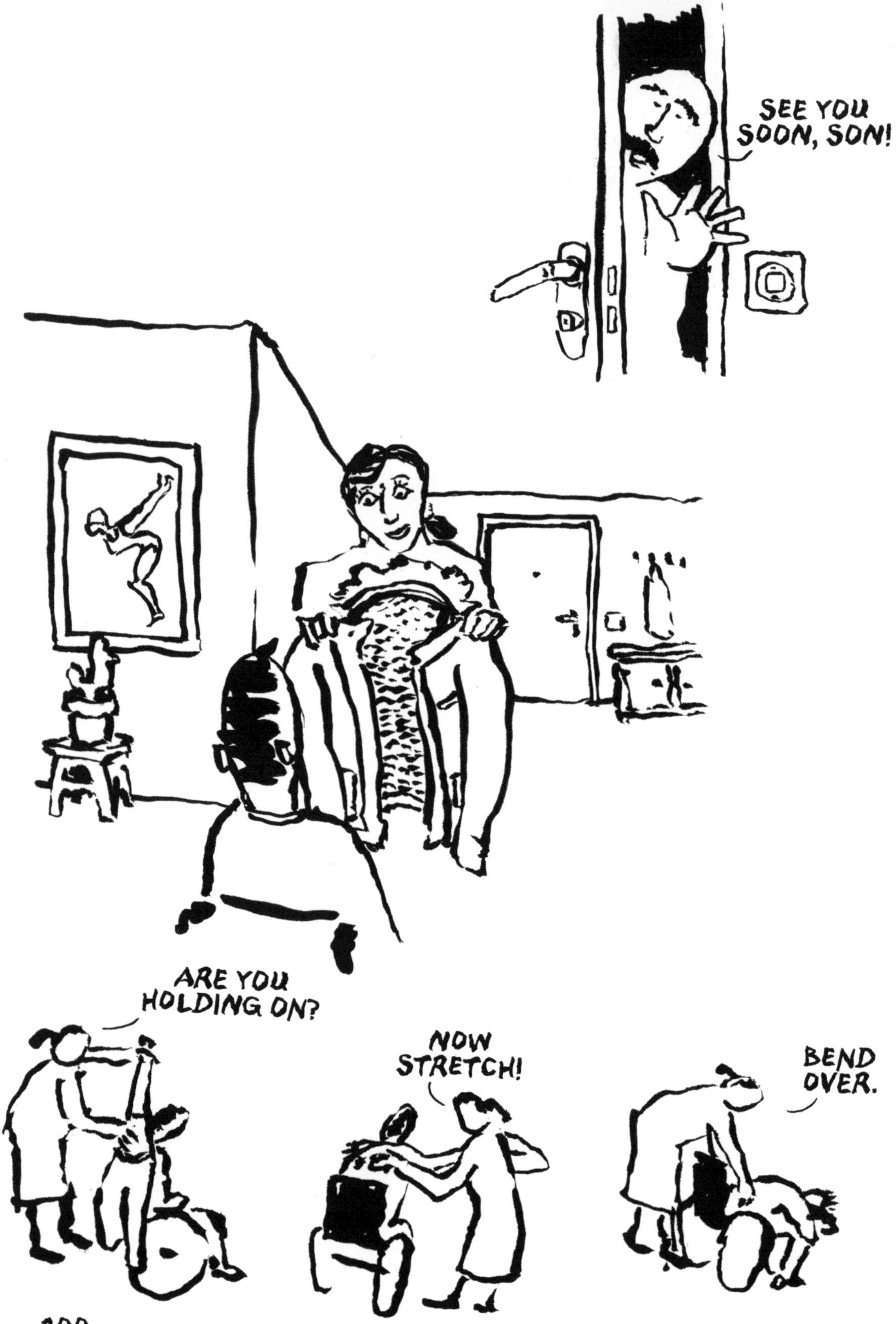
SEE YOU SOON, SON!
ARE YOU HOLDING ON?
NOW STRETCH!
BEND OVER.

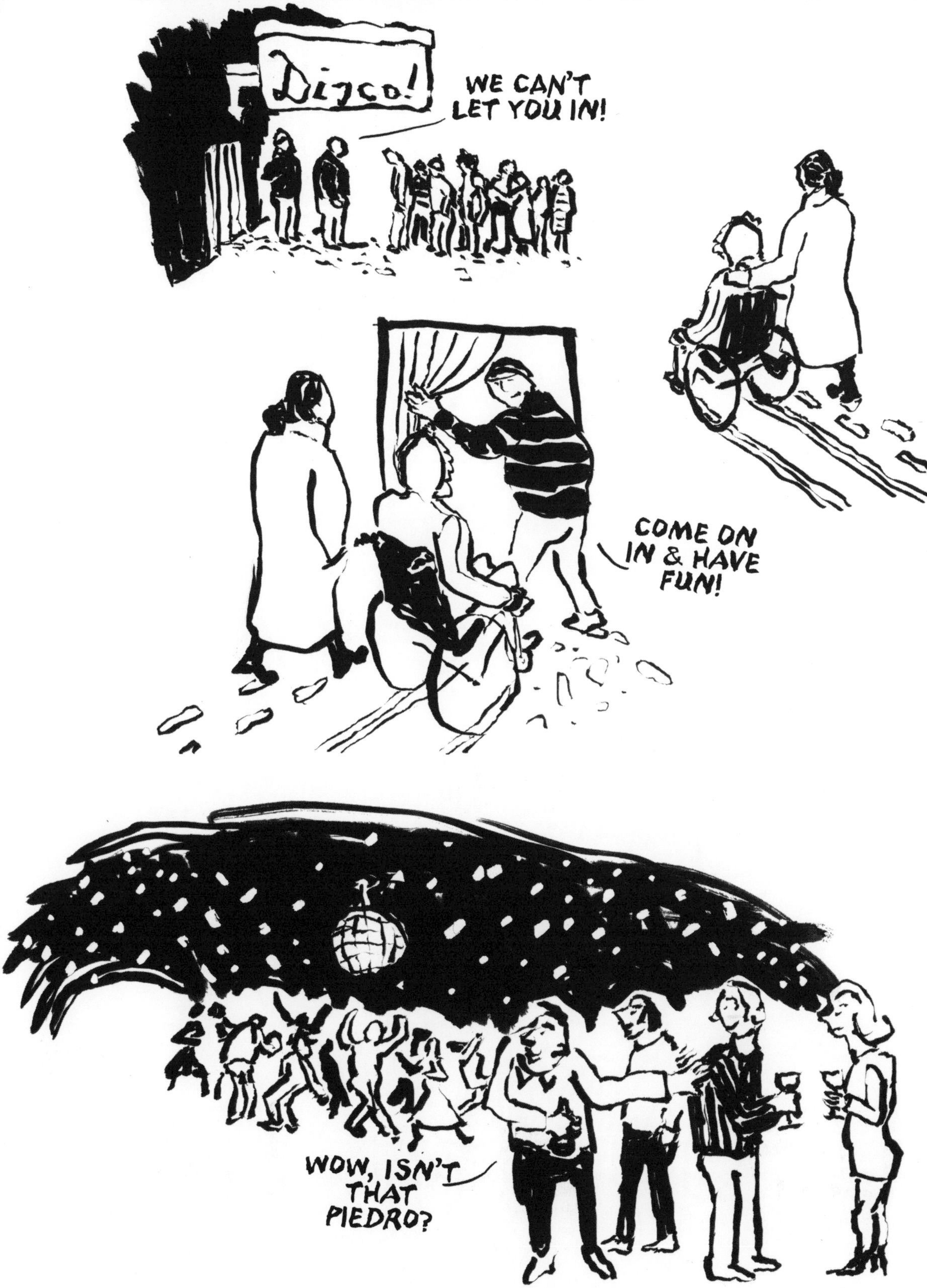
WE CAN'T LET YOU IN!
COME ON IN & HAVE FUN!
WOW, ISN'T THAT PIEDRO?

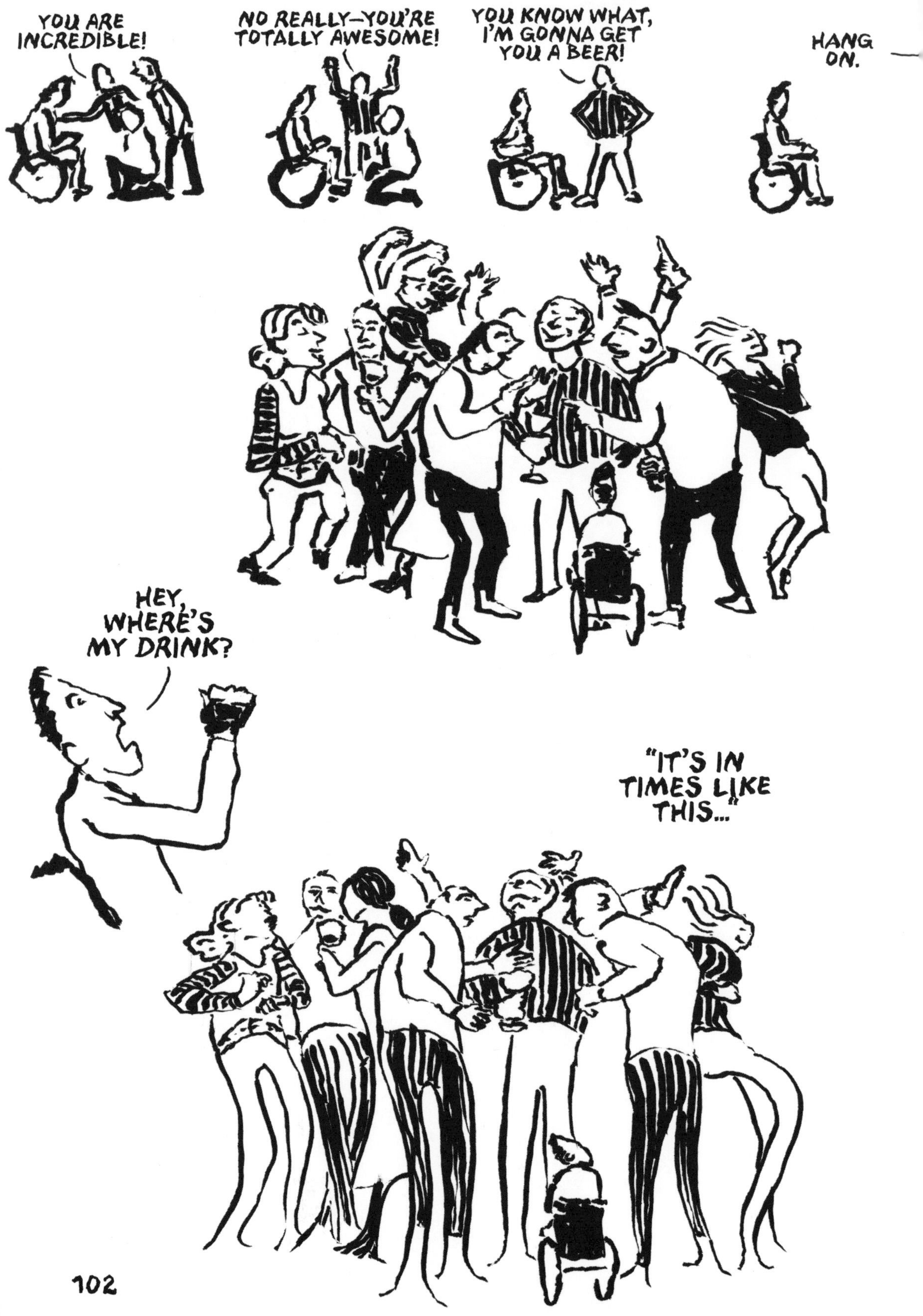
YOU ARE INCREDIBLE!
NO REALLY—YOU'RE TOTALLY AWESOME!
YOU KNOW WHAT, I'M GONNA GET YOU A BEER!
HANG ON.
HEY, WHERE'S MY DRINK?
"IT'S IN TIMES LIKE THIS..."

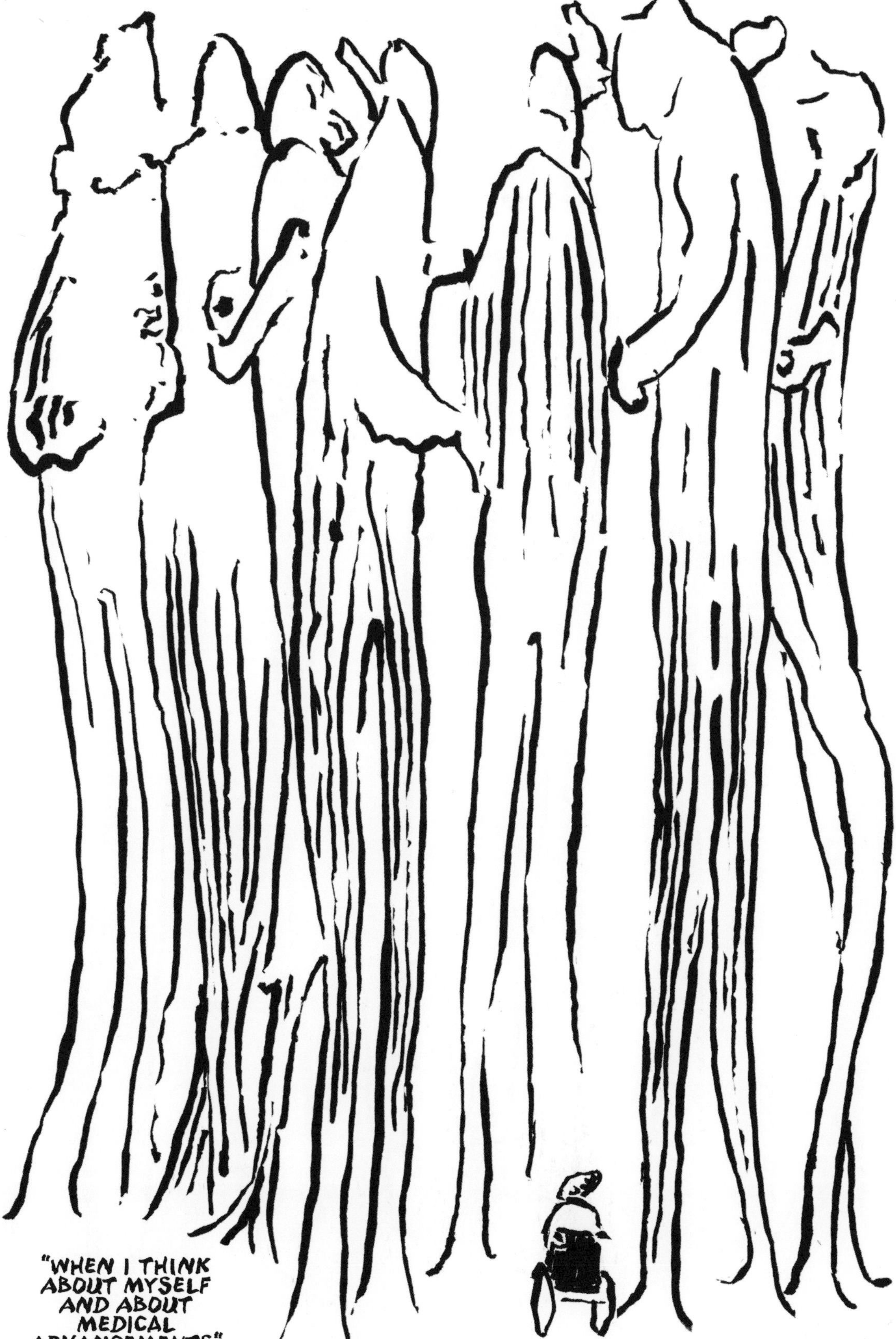
"WHEN I THINK
ABOUT MYSELF
AND ABOUT
MEDICAL
ADVANCEMENTS"

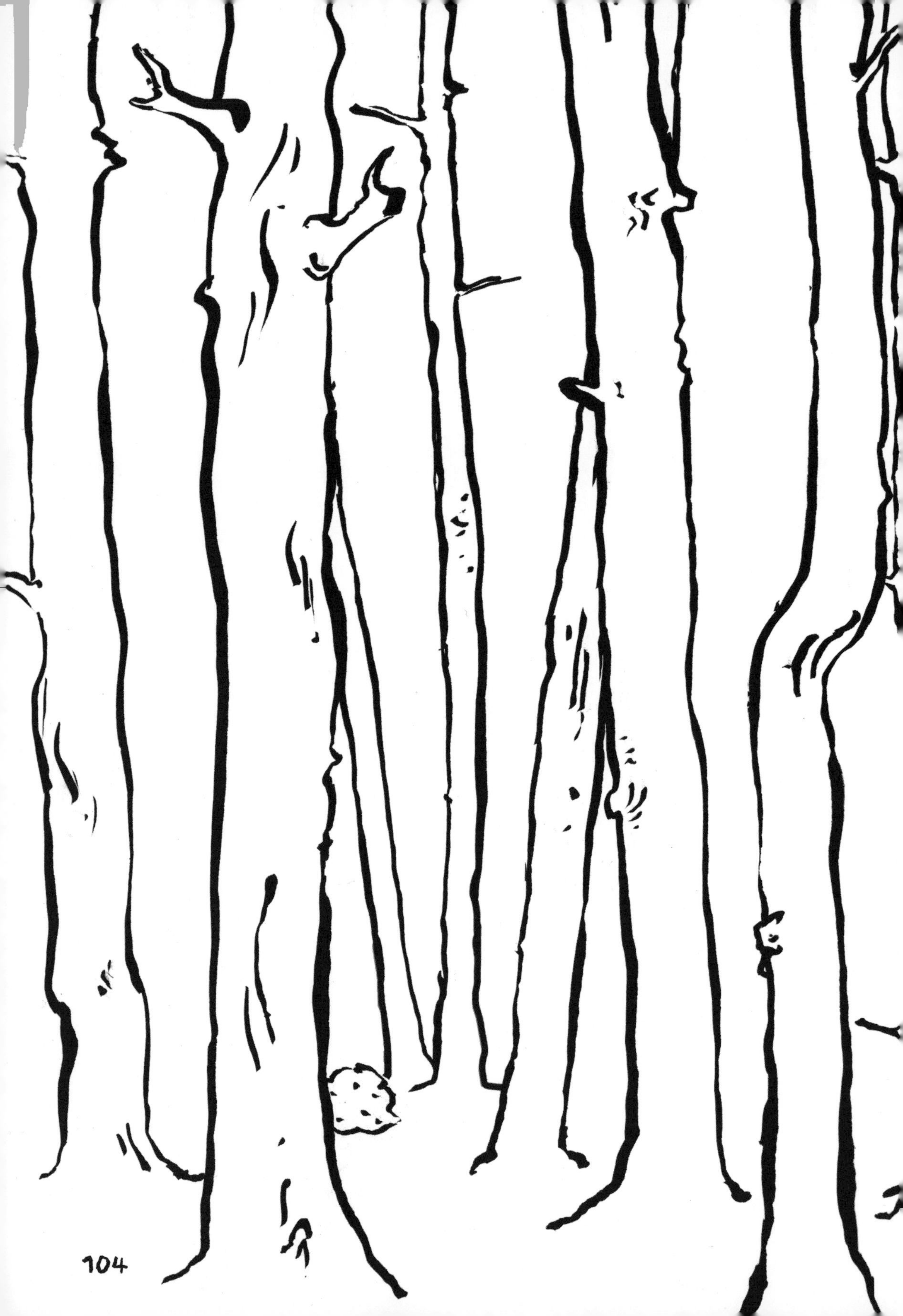

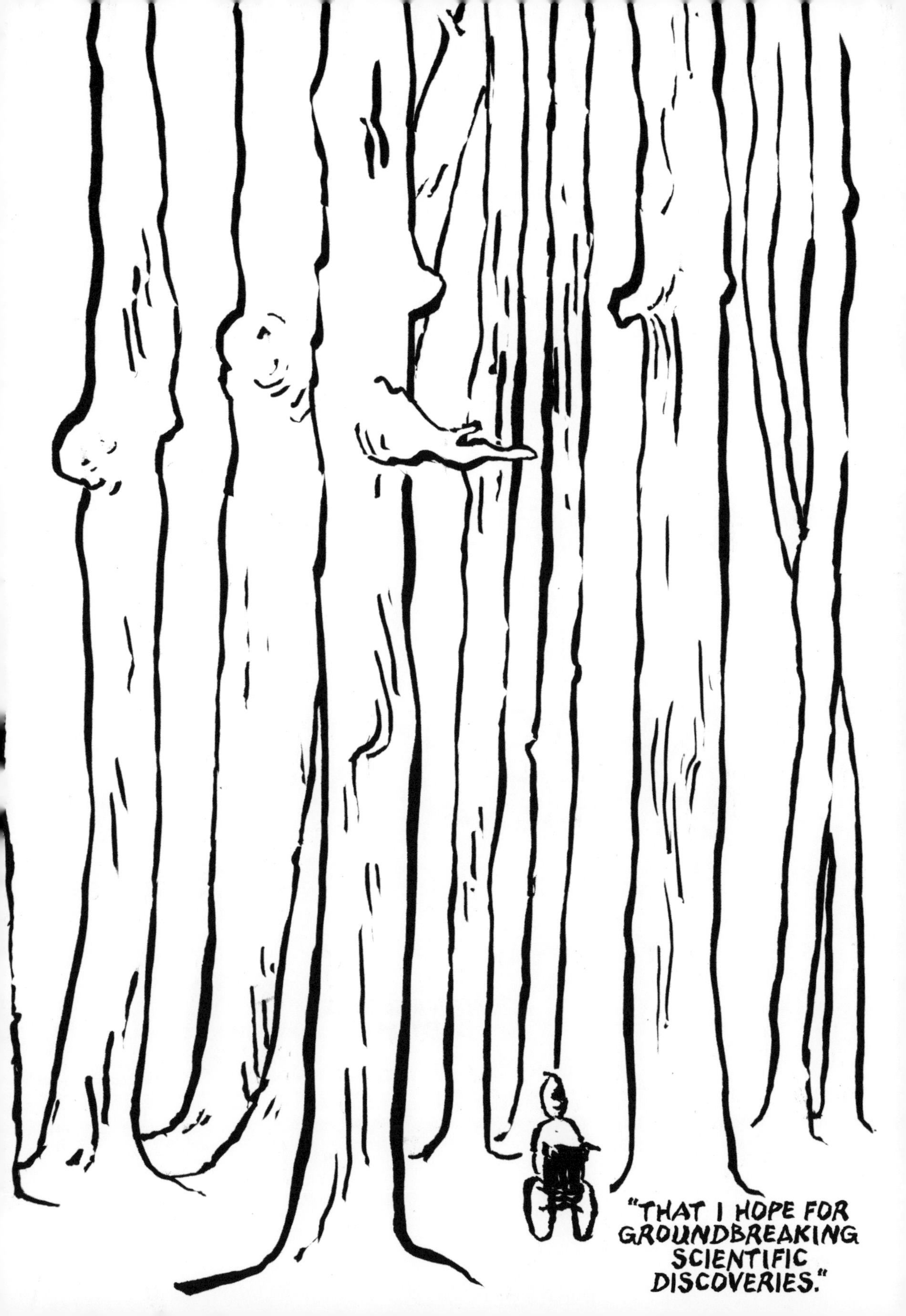
"THAT I HOPE FOR GROUNDBREAKING SCIENTIFIC DISCOVERIES."

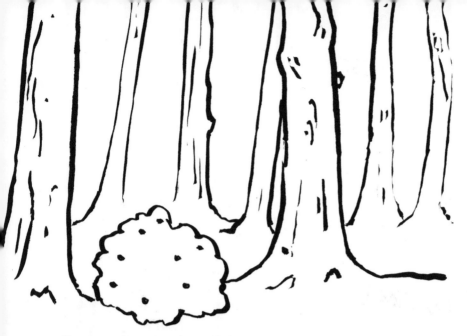

"OR THE INVENTION OF A MIRACLE DRUG."

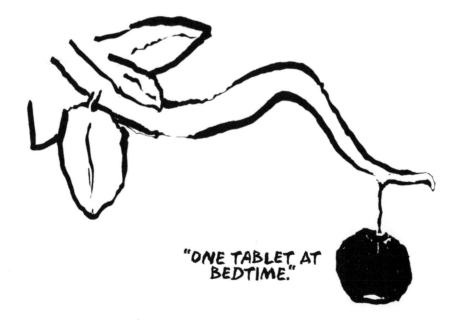

"ONE TABLET AT BEDTIME."

"TAKE IT WITH A SIP OF WATER."

"THEN JUST WAIT FOR IT TO DO ITS WORK."

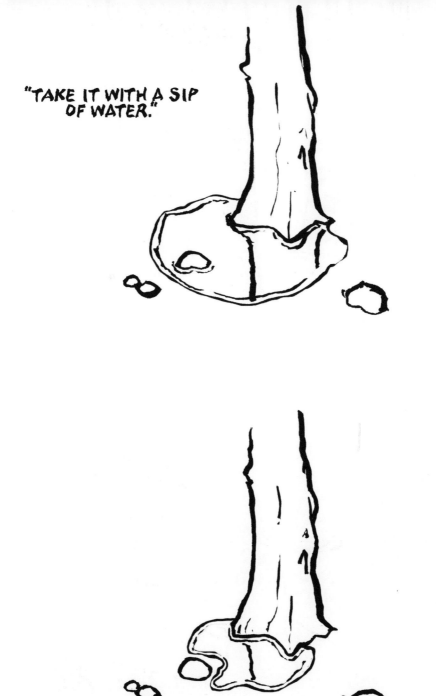

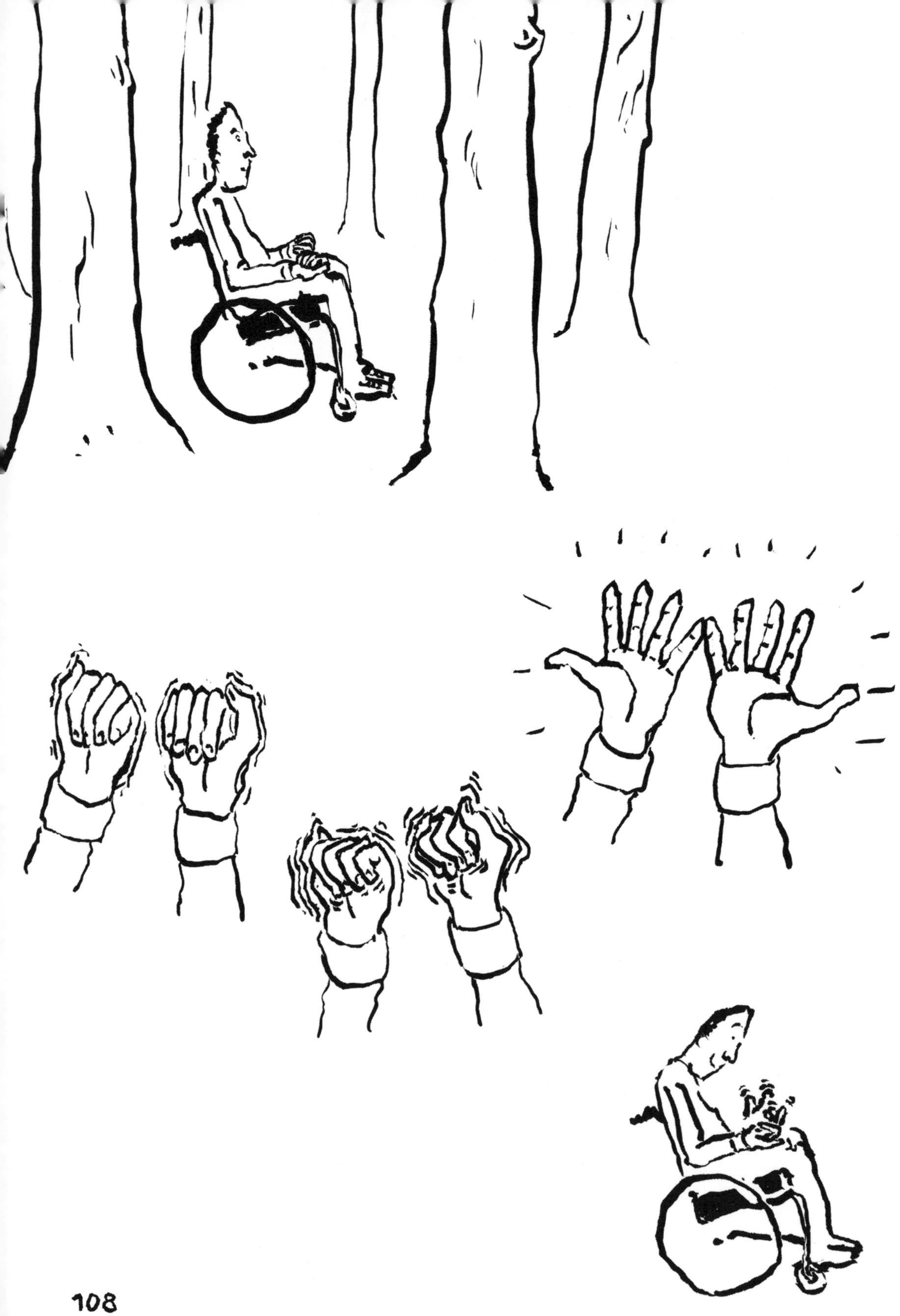

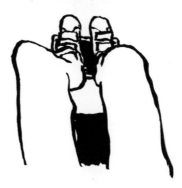

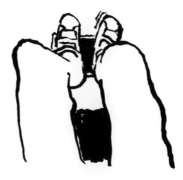

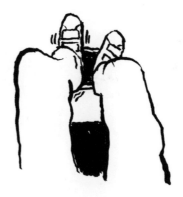

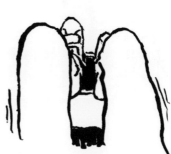

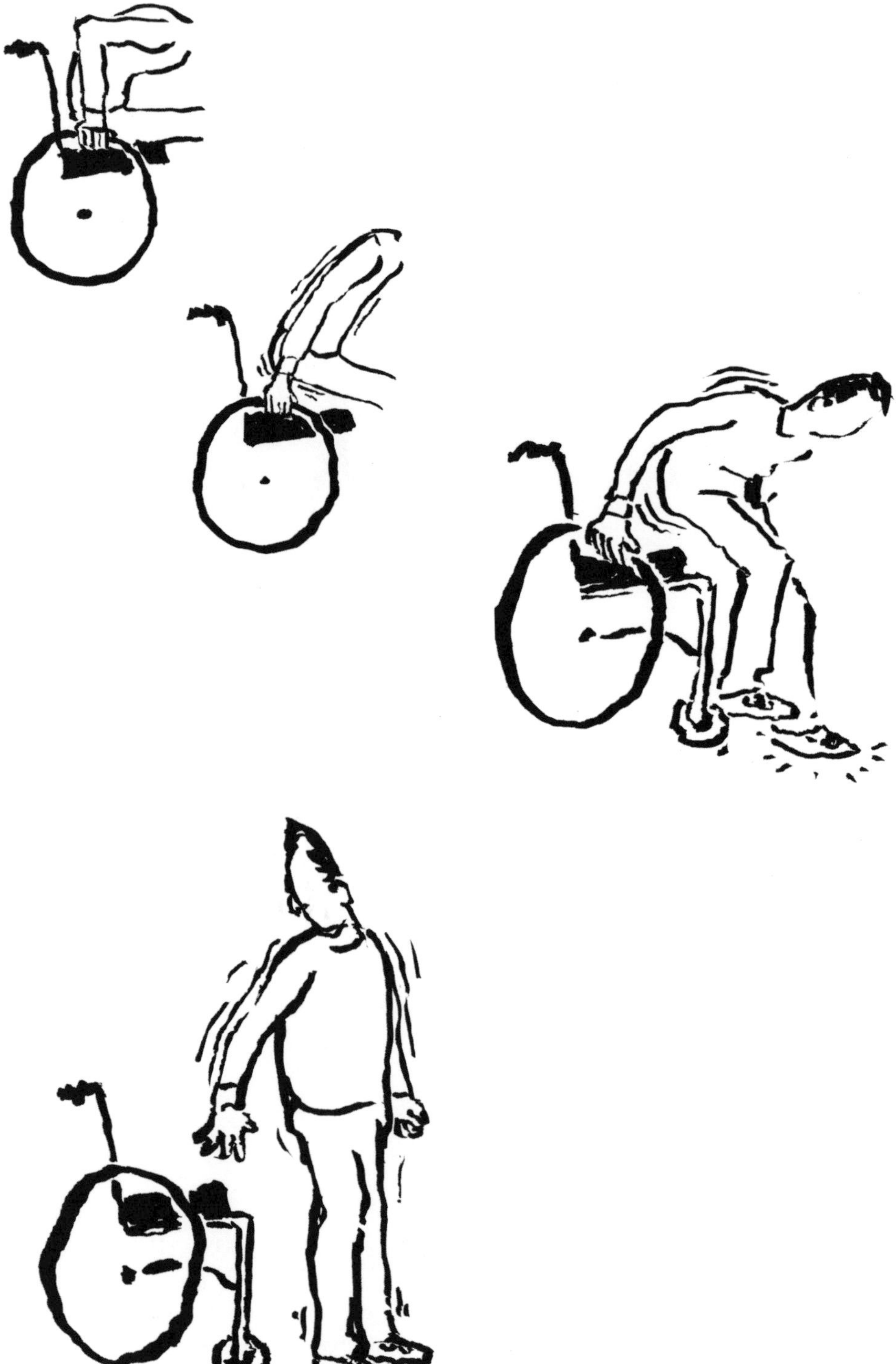

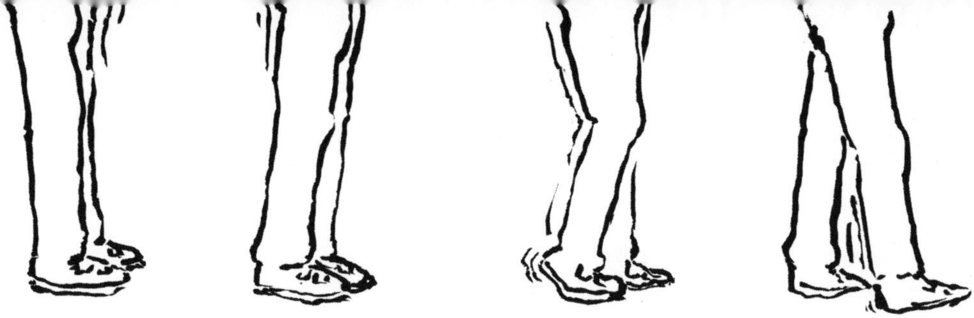

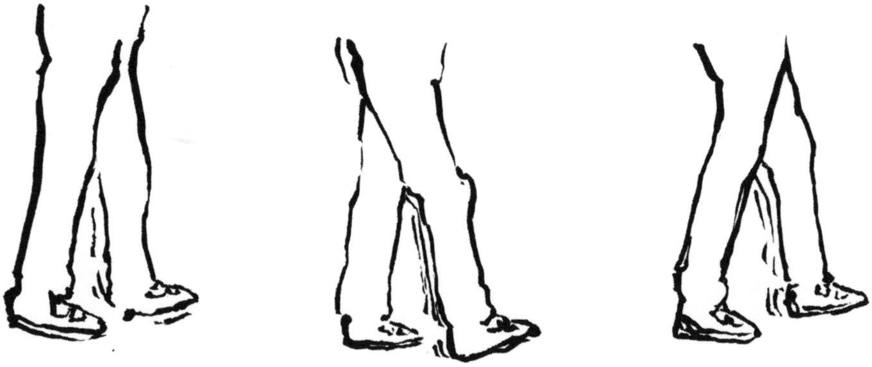

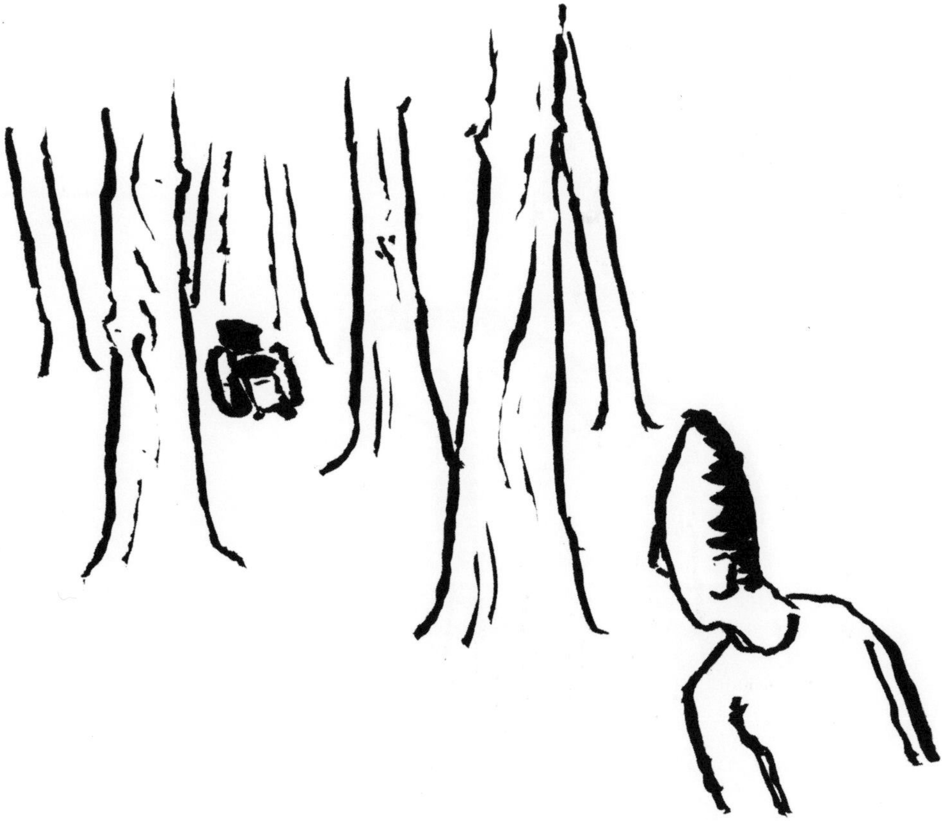

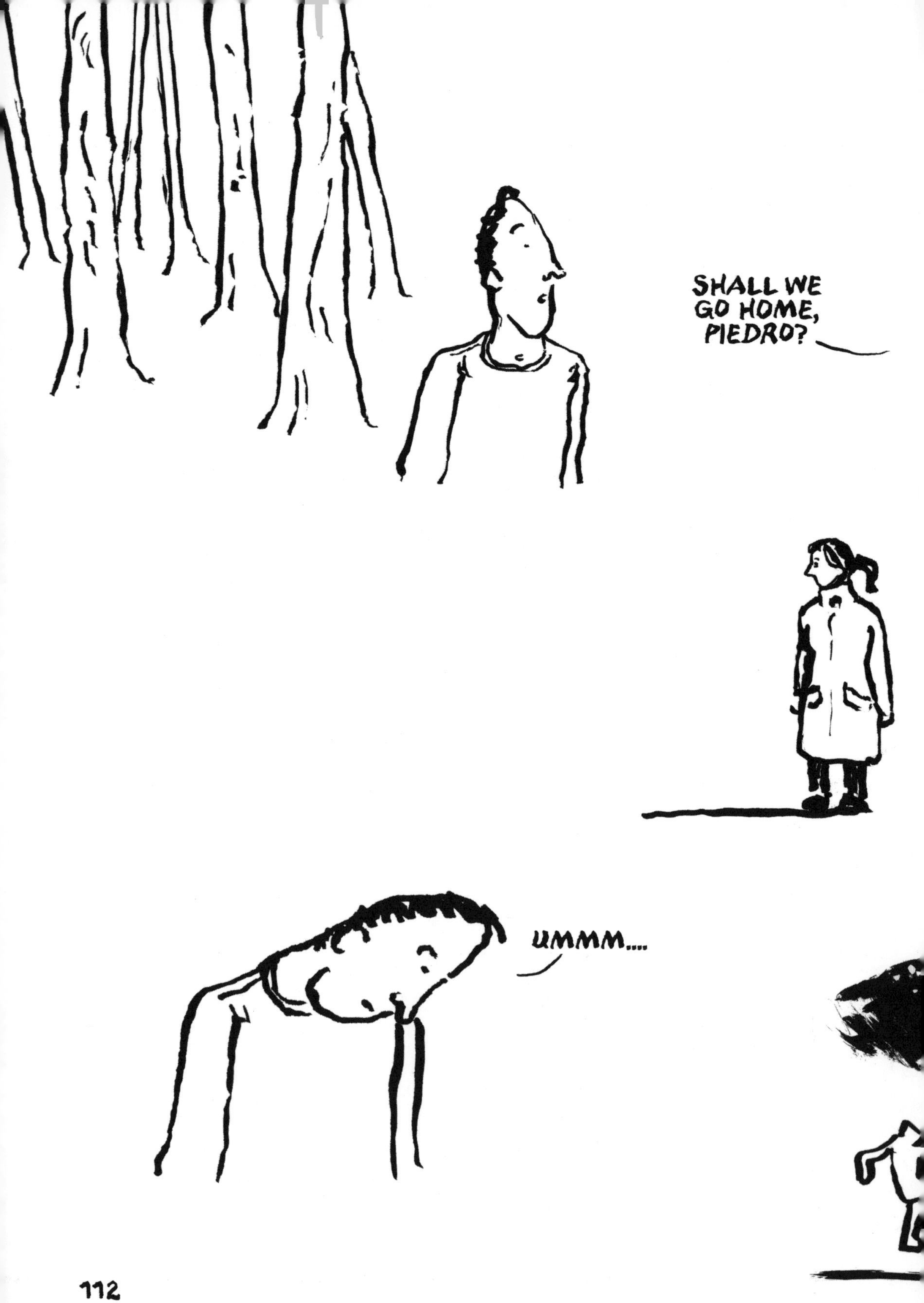
SHALL WE GO HOME, PIEDRO?
UMMM....

ALREADY ON MY WAY, CHARLOTTE.

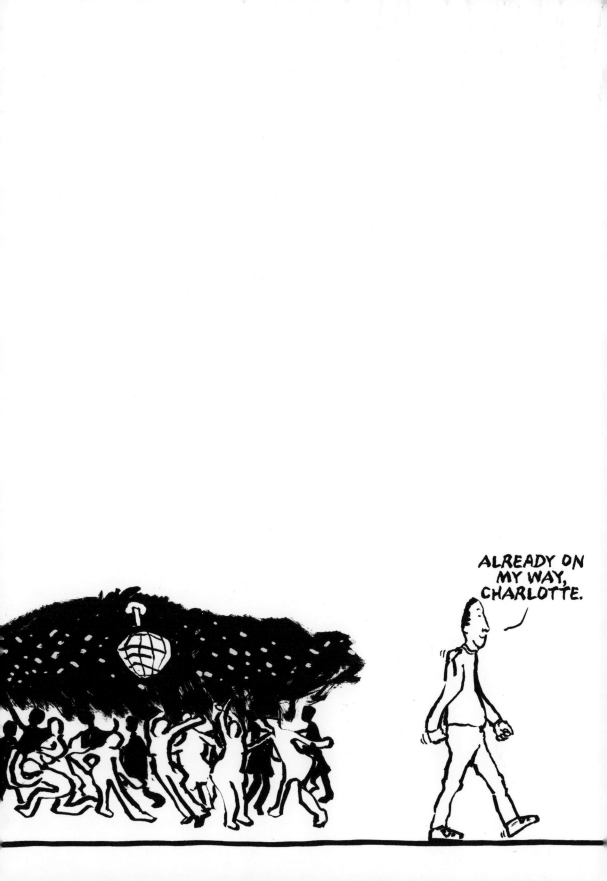

The translation of this work was supported by a grant from the Goethe-Institut in the framework of the Books First program.

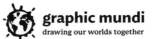

GOETHE INSTITUT

Library of Congress Cataloging-in-Publication Data

Names: Burkart, Roland (Artist), author, illustrator. | Hoffmeyer, Natascha, translator.
Title: Twister / Roland Burkart ; translated by Natascha Hoffmeyer.
Other titles: Wirbelsturm. English
Description: University Park, Pennsylvania : The Pennsylvania State University Press, [2020] | "Originally published as Wirbelsturm, ©2017, Edition Moderne, Switzerland."
Summary: "A fictionalized narrative, in graphic novel format, of the author's experiences as a quadriplegic following injuries he sustained from an accident"—Provided by publisher.
Identifiers: LCCN 2020028355 | ISBN 9780271088082 (paperback)
Subjects: LCSH: Quadriplegics—Comic books, strips, etc. | LCGFT: Graphic novels.
Classification: LCC PN6790.S93 B8713 2020 | DDC 741.5/9494—dc23
LC record available at https://lccn.loc.gov/2020028355

Printed in China
Published by The Pennsylvania State University Press, University Park, PA 16802-1003

Translated by Natascha Hoffmeyer

Originally published as *Wirbelsturm*

graphic mundi
drawing our worlds together

Graphic Mundi is an imprint of The Pennsylvania State University Press.

The Pennsylvania State University Press is a member of the Association of University Presses.

It is the policy of The Pennsylvania State University Press to use acid-free paper. Publications on uncoated stock satisfy the minimum requirements of American National Standard for Information Sciences—Permanence of Paper for Printed Library Material, ANSI Z39.48–1992.

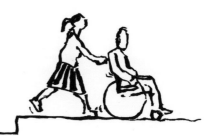

DEC - 7 2021